SPLASH INTO CALM

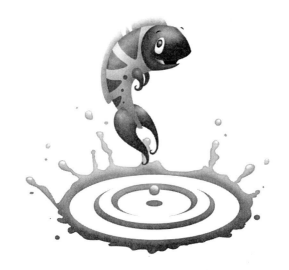

Ellen Sichel

Splash Into Calm:
Custom Calm Chronicles

Copyright© 2012 Ellen Sichel. All rights reserved. No part of this book may be reproduced or reprinted in any form or by any means, electronic or mechanical, including photocopying, recording, or by any information storage and retrieval system, without permission in writing from the publisher.

For information regarding permission to reprint material from this book, please mail or email your request to: Ellen@CustomCalm.com

PO Box 76396
Atlanta, GA 30358
CustomCalm.com

Author: Ellen Sichel
Project Manager: Bonnie Daneker of Write Advisors, LLC
Illustrator: Jamie Sichel
Author Photo: Bill Adler Photography ™
Book Design: Debbie Kerr of Office Angels
Copy Editor: Judy Usherson of Office Angels
Logo Design: Alliene Bouchard

Sichel, Ellen
Splash Into Calm; Custom Calm Chronicles/ Ellen Sichel
Foreword by Christy Andrews
ISBN 978-0-9859664-0-9
1. Personal growth 2. Stress management 3. Pain management
Manufactured in the United States of America
Cover Design: Jamie Sichel
Printed in the United States of America by: BookLogix®, Alpharetta, Georgia

∞ This paper meets the requirements of ANSI/NISO Z39.48-1992 (Permanence of Paper)

Dedication

To those living with chronic stress,
pain and illness who choose to live life to the fullest.
Their courage, tenacity and willingness to change
inspire me on a daily basis.

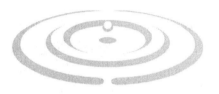

CUSTOM CALM

Table of Contents

Foreword	vii
Acknowledgements	ix
Introduction	xi

January Theme: New Beginnings

Week 1 - Resolutions	17
Week 2 - Progress, Not Perfection	21
Week 3 - Change	25
Week 4 - Motivation for Change: Gary's Story	29

February Theme: Love & Kindness

Week 5 - Compassion	35
Week 6 - The Ultimate Valentine's Gift	39
Week 7 - We Are All Divine	43
Week 8 - Heart Health	47

March Theme: Pain & Illness

Week 9 - Awareness	53
Week 10 - Acceptance	57
Week 11 - Community	61
Week 12 - Empowerment	65

April Theme: Emergence

Week 13 - Lighten Up!	73
Week 14 - Easter and Passover	77
Week 15 - Emergence from Workaholism: Shellie's Story	81
Week 16 - Live in Truth	85

May Theme: Travel

Week 17 - Vacation Time	91
Week 18 - Impact of Travel: The Body	95
Week 19 - Impact of Travel: The Mind	99
Week 20 - Enjoy the Journey	103

June Theme: Balanced Living

Week 21 - Activity	109
Week 22 - Living Life Fully	113
Week 23 - Sleep	117

Week 24 - Balance from the Inside-Out: Diane's Story   123

July Theme: Relationships & Emotions
Week 25 - Un-Hook from Reaction   129
Week 26 - Personality Traits   133
Week 27 - Communication   137
Week 28 - Worry or Grace   141

August Theme: Perspective
Week 29 - Intuition and Meditation   147
Week 30 - Freedom to Choose   151
Week 31 – Attitude of Gratitude   157
Week 32 - That's Life: Jamie's Story   161

September Theme: Responsibility
Week 33 - Self Care   167
Week 34 - Health Challenges of Loved Ones   171
Week 35 - Caregiving for Elders   175
Week 36 –Responsibility Equals Freedom   181

October Theme: Day-to-Day Living
Week 37 - Simple Pleasures   187
Week 38 - Household Duties   191
Week 39 - Habits   195
Week 40 - Procrastination   199

November Theme: Digestion
Week 41 - Food Glorious Food   205
Week 42 - Thanksgiving   209
Week 43 - Cultivating Attitudes   215
Week 44 - Digesting Life: Dana's Story   219

December Theme: Stress
Week 45 - Enjoy the Holiday Season   225
Week 46 - The Truth about Stress   229
Week 47 - Ride the Waves: Grey's Story   235
Week 48 - Splash into Calm   239

Bibliography   243
About the Author   249

Foreword

The book you are holding in your hand has the potential to change your life. I know this because I've had the privilege of having a front row seat to the power of Ellen Sichel's messages for almost a decade. I've watched from afar as she individually guides cancer patients through classes to help them manage their treatment and reduce stress. And I've experienced her wisdom personally, as well. I'll never forget bemoaning how a recent family vacation didn't live up to my expectations. She took my shoulder and simply pointed out, "*That's because we all take ourselves on vacation with us. We show up to vacation the way we show up to life.*" Those wise words made such an impression on me and I know I'll never approach another family vacation the same way.

When I first met Ellen at the Cancer Support Community Atlanta I was told that she truly believes that what she teaches can change the world. As I began to watch her work and saw her interact with each cancer patient we serve at our facility, I saw that little by little, she was changing *everyone's* world. The ripple effect of Ellen grew and soon our facility was abuzz about this new instructor whose bag of tricks reached far wider than a simple wellness class.

As so often happens in our serendipitous world, Ellen's initial participation here was not part of a big plan. She came to us as a substitute yoga instructor for just a few classes and almost immediately her magic began to be felt. As our participants experienced her unique methods of teaching and all she could offer, they begged for more of her. Years later, her repertoire at CSC Atlanta continues to grow, as does her fan base, reaching way beyond our community.

Just as Ellen came to us in a serendipitous way, your journey with Ellen's teaching might also have happened by chance. Perhaps you simply ran across this book at a local store and were intrigued by the cover. In whatever way you've come upon *Splash Into Calm,* consider the pages you hold in your hand a gift that can help you change your approach to so many areas of your life—how you manage pain and illness, how to react and appreciate the difference in others, even how to be a better listener. Treat yourself to a weekly dedication of time with *Splash Into Calm* and you'll find significant changes happening in your life. Who knows? You might even find yourself looking forward to family vacations again!

Christy Andrews
Executive Director
Cancer Support Community – Atlanta

Acknowledgements

I must begin with my husband and his unwavering love, support, and encouragement for all that I want to achieve. My children, Jennifer and Jamie, have been my teachers and much of this book comes as a result of our lives together.

My parents and grandmother always taught me that I could do whatever I set my mind to. I am forever grateful for that lesson. My mother helped and inspired me every step of the way through her caring and total confidence in my abilities. My sister is my cheering squad, and my brothers help me keep my sense of humor.

My project manager, Bonnie Daneker of Write Advisors, has been with me every step of the way. Her clear guidance, deadlines, and encouragement have transformed my many ideas into a book and I am forever grateful for her professionalism and vision.

There were seven contributors who generously offered their stories. I thank them for their honesty and inspiration: Shellie Kirk; Diane Mitchel; Dana Zahn; Grey Duddleston; Jamie Sichel, who is a professional illustrator (she created the character and designs throughout this book); and Dr. Gary Bodner, who is also a professional painter (Gary's beautiful work can be seen in different galleries throughout the Southeast including Anne Irwin Fine Art Gallery in Atlanta. He was named Southeast Painter of the Year in 2011.) Jennifer Sichel graciously granted me permission to share her story.

As with any first book, there are so many in the past that have influenced the words on the pages. There have been teachers, institutions, friends and clients along the way and the list is too long to mention them all—I sincerely thank you. Here are a few that I am compelled to mention:

Cancer Support Community Atlanta; Duke University Integrative Medicine; Plum Tree Yoga; Master Yoga Foundation; Jon Kabat-Zinn; Kashi Foundation and the philanthropic teachings of the recently-deceased Ma Jaya Sati Bhagavati; Camp

Fernwood; Alliene Bouchard, who guided me in conceptualizing my logo design; and Jay Solomon and Eszter Boda of More of Me to Love, who planted the seed for a book years back.

I am deeply grateful for all of you. You have helped inspire me to live the work I teach.

Introduction

Calm living—it seems it like a nice concept, but in today's stressful world, is it realistic?

My experience is yes, it is possible for every one of us to enjoy a relaxed way of being. First, I need to explain what I mean by calm living, and then you will realize that you can be the beneficiary of a richer, more nourishing life.

Calm living gives you the ability to embrace each moment of your day. It opens you up to increased joy, spontaneity, and pleasure because you are aware and alert.

I am not implying that you will not have stress in your life, because that would be unrealistic. Stress is a fact of life, even during wonderful times. The key is to know how to respond to a stressful situation. I wrote this book because I wanted to share my approach to this universal challenge. This book gives you the ability to bring yourself back to your center without stress taking over.

Most clients I consult have busy lives and want to enjoy themselves, yet they are affected by the consequences of stress. You do not have to give up your full life in order to live calmly. You can have it all—being calm and full of energy.

I realized early on in my work that it is vital to meet people where they are. In this complex world, there is a need for simplicity. That is exactly what this book is about—simple, realistic practices and ideas that profoundly enhance your daily living. I have chosen to communicate in a more personal manner, with lightness, sharing my own experiences as well as those of my clients—as if we were sitting together chatting.

Many practices and concepts in this book are based on yoga traditions comprising breathing practices, meditation, yoga stretches, and many other centering techniques (focusing awareness so you can attain a calm state). While there might be an air of granola (my friend calls it "la-di-da") surrounding yoga and meditation, I assure you that it not "new age" or "alternative" but complementary to that which is available in the medical profession. Not only have yoga and centering practices been around since the dawn of time, but now hospitals, universities, and doctors are investing time and money on research and evidence that support its value. My colleagues and I have the challenge of being taken seriously because we are not doctors, nor do we have advanced degrees. What we do have is years of hands-on experience, education, and the depth of understanding that can only be gained by living and breathing what we teach. I am thrilled and grateful to have access to the extensive knowledge and training of the medical profession and the many universities and governmental entities whose research supports these practices.

In keeping with simplicity, I have designed an easy-to-follow format for this book. It is based on the calendar year and presented in monthly themes, each having four articles. You can read one per week, skip around to the theme on which you need some insight or read the entire book at a pace that works for you. It is just that easy. The topics are as follows:

January:	New Beginnings
February:	Love & Kindness
March:	Pain & Illness
April:	Emergence
May:	Travel
June:	Balanced Living
July:	Relationships & Emotions
August:	Perspective
September:	Responsibility
October:	Day-to-Day Living
November:	Digestion
December:	Stress

These themes are universal, regardless of age, gender, profession, or location. As you read the articles and splash around in the techniques, keep in mind that they are designed for you—in both your personal and professional life. My premise is simple: *if they work for me, they will work for you.*

Enjoy the book—I had a great time writing it!

Warm Regards,

Eileen

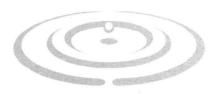

CUSTOM CALM

JANUARY

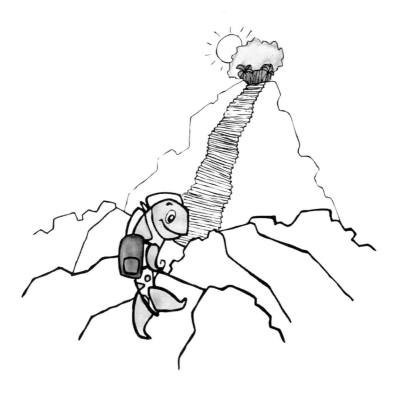

New Beginnings

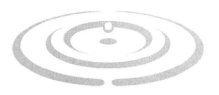

CUSTOM CALM

WEEK ONE

RESOLUTIONS

Welcome to *Custom Calm Chronic*les. This year, join me and discover how to splash into calm. No bathing suit is needed, no special gear—that would be too much work. *Custom Calm Chronicles* keep things easy, uplifting, and, most of all, practical. All you need is a bit of curiosity and a few minutes each week. Then you'll be able to splash around in the uplifting possibilities inherent in the joy of calm living.

January is a great time to begin. The holiday season is now behind us and we are off to a fresh start. January is when we take time to reflect, reevaluate priorities, set goals, and make changes. We refer to this custom as New Year's Resolutions. Some people refuse to do this as they have fallen off the New Year's Resolutions wagon once too often. Others, those who have not given up hope, set goals, feel motivated, and are ready to begin.

With or without formal New Year's Resolutions, we all have the sincere desire to improve our lives in some way. We might begin a diet, exercise, join a class, or get organized, but something derails us. We get off to a strong start, but sooner or later our good intentions peter out and before we know it we are back to our old habits and behaviors.

Let's take a look at some of the culprits. First of all, the common activities I have listed above are not exactly enjoyable or enticing. Let's sweeten the pot of success and make our goals seem less daunting and more manageable and realistic—let's choose an avenue that will ensure success.

Take a moment and think: is there anything specific you want to improve in your life? My experience has been that to succeed, intention is not enough. It takes more than just wanting to do it—any kind of improvement takes commitment and practice. These are not my favorite words. When I was a kid, my mother thought it would be nice for me to learn piano (not her best idea). She told me I had to practice the scales every day, which I did. I quickly realized, however, that I disliked piano and soon quit.

As I got older, I again had to practice, this time to get my driver's license. My license spelled *freedom* to me, so it was worth the commitment of my time. I made the arrangements to practice daily and finally, after the third try, I got my license. Yes, it seems that I needed a bit more commitment to improve my three-point turns and parallel parking! My commitment and practice helped me overcome failure.

Think about something you started but didn't finish. Then think about the experience of beginning something challenging that you stuck with until completion. What was the difference? Practice, consistency, and devotion were fundamental to your success.

There is a teaching in yoga that addresses this. It tells us that practice needs to be firmly established by being continued for a long time, without interruption, and with devotion.

You might be thinking, "Oh great, it's hard enough to practice, and now I have to practice for a long time? I want to just magically be able to get in shape, become computer literate, and learn a new language."

I agree.

At the start of the New Year you made a resolution to do something that is certain to improve the quality of your life. We've talked about three ingredients for success: intention, commitment, and practice. So, allow me take it a step further. You need to combine these ingredients to create structure until it forms a habit.

There are many opinions of how long it takes to establish a habit, but consistency and repetition are key elements. Include a practice in your daily schedule (assuming you look at your schedule) so it is part of your activities. Practice every day—whether you want to or not. If you wait for the feeling to come, you will wait a long time. Action is the key. It's like the Nike ad: *Just do it!*

I admit, this still does not sound very enticing, so I have saved the best ingredient for last—an important one that is often neglected: devotion. Devotion reframes our attitude toward our resolution, which in turn impacts the results.

Let's take a look at the word *devotion*. Devotion is often thought of as dedication and loyalty, or having selfless affection toward another. It seems so much easier to devote ourselves to others. When you hear the term "devoted" to describe spouse, parent, child, teacher, or employee, what does it bring to mind? Loving. Always willing to be there. Kind. Dedicated. Each of us has one or more of these attributes.

Imagine if you could give this same devotion to yourself? The loyalty and dedication I am speaking about is the devotion toward feeling good—the devotion toward you. When approaching your resolutions, treat yourself with the same kindness and patience you would give a child learning to walk. You would never yell at your child for falling. There is a learning curve to everything new, so be consistent and hang in there!

I know treating yourself with kindness and patience is extremely challenging for some of us. If that is the case, then why not make treating yourself with kindness your resolution? Devotion to yourself will not only improve your physical well-being, but will enhance other aspects of your life, including your relationships.

Your attitude about the changes you are working toward will affect your success. When you try to force yourself to do something or even put a guilt trip on yourself, you will become as resistant as a rebellious child. Think about the response of a two-year-old when you want them to do something: a resounding NO! A softer, caring voice, devoted to your own welfare and happiness is much more inviting.

Give yourself permission to experience the ups and downs of new resolutions. The quality of your entire life will change; I guarantee it.

This week, give these a try:

- Make your resolution very approachable and realistic, so you can actually work on making it happen.
- Schedule the time on your calendar to focus on whatever it is that you are trying to change. It is best to schedule this practice at the same time each day or week.
- If it is behavior you're changing, then leave little written reminders. For example, if you are trying to drink more water leave a note in an obvious place.
- Be consistent.
- Cultivate a mindset of devotion to yourself with kind reminders.
- Be careful of your mind coming up with creative excuses.
- No matter how small a success you've had on following through, congratulate yourself. It's a big deal!

These suggestions might seem incredibly simple, but I assure you they will set you up for success. Your New Year will be off to a great beginning and the momentum will continue. Remember, it will take time for your resolutions to become a part of your daily life. And even if you do not have any resolutions, you can benefit from more devotion to yourself. If you have already fallen off the New Year's Resolution Wagon, hop back on, dust yourself off, and read the next entry!

WEEK TWO

PROGRESS, NOT PERFECTION

Let's expand on Week One's topic of setting ourselves up for continued success with our resolutions. I am sure, even with our energetic start and new-found self-devotion, we will naturally waver and wonder if our effort is worth the results we hope to attain.

Often people ask me: "Will this work?" and I confidently reply: "Yes, if you do it!" Then I add, "You will probably need a bit more inspiration to keep your momentum going." The following quote by Susan Smith Jones, PhD, seems quite fitting: "Discipline is the ability to carry out a resolution long after the mood has left you."

Having intention and resolve is a great start and will probably sustain you for a short time, but we need follow-through and discipline. (Sorry if that word brings back unpleasant memories!) Discipline is misunderstood as something punishing, rigid, and unwavering. Actually, it really implies that there is some kind of skill, activity, or routine that we want to develop or improve upon. Think of the early painting apprentices. They used discipline to learn the skill from the Masters; it wasn't always fun but they stuck to it.

Let's take this notion a bit further. While it is true that to attain success on your resolution you need discipline, there is another element that will encourage success: perseverance. What we want to avoid is giving up; instead, we want to follow through. Joseph P. Kennedy advised, "When the going gets tough, the tough get going." The challenge is how to stay the course when you want to back off and give up.

Here are a few concepts that will give you the boost needed when you face such challenges or resistance:

- The first priority is to focus on attaining your goal *one day at a time,* or even one minute at a time. Putting one foot in front of the other will avoid overwhelm and frustration on the long road ahead. All progress is good progress.
- Keep your goal in mind without getting caught up in it. When your mind kicks in with excuses or distractions, it is harmful for achieving your goals. When your mind tells you: "You can skip today, no big deal" or "I don't have the time to practice" or "Is it really worth the hassle?" or "Well, I skipped yesterday, so why bother—I have already failed," it's easy to think of yourself as a loser. Here is my personal favorite: "I am too out of shape and old to do this." Of course that is the very reason you are doing it! It comes down to this: We need to keep our minds on track because our thoughts can sabotage any progress.

The following points must be practiced simultaneously so you can stay in balance:

- Be persistent and steady with your practice to make any headway. When you center your attention on staying consistent, you will set yourself up for success because your focus is on what is right in front of you.
- Persistence alone will set you up for becoming too rigid with the process, so you want to couple it with letting go of the outcome of your actions. This is important because it is easy to get caught in the cycle of "doing it right" which encourages perfectionism. Continue to remain consistent with your progress and do not worry about your desired outcome.

Establishing a habit (which we referred to in Week One) will propel your progress. I needed to do this while writing this book, otherwise I would have quit long ago. I remember when I began; I could feel my heart quicken and breath shorten. I almost fell off my chair when my editor gave me the timeline! But I established a daily writing practice, while giving myself permission to take needed breaks. This steady process enabled me to reach my goal. I kept my goal in sight, without fixating on it. The process of feeling some sense of accomplishment will inspire you, so from time to time take a look back and see how far you have come.

Some important tips:

- Record your progress, any progress.
- If you miss a day and your mind starts to derail you, take a few breaths and tell yourself: "Just for today, I will do this practice." That will keep you in the moment and away from the enormity of the goal.
- The next day, tell yourself: "Just for today, I will do this practice." Do this every time you need to practice and you will build momentum. Stay focused on the task at hand, not the end result.
- Each day when you finish, take a slow deep breath and tell yourself, "Good job!"

If you are working some kind of centering practice like adding meditation to your routine, try these suggestions too:

- Find a space in your home or office and make it inviting and comfortable. This is important for anything you need to accomplish, especially when working for hours on the computer.

- Create a ritual: We all have rituals—things we do consistently that works for us, like morning rituals and bedtime rituals. Remember to set up a time each day and do your practice, even if your mind is giving you reason not to—and it will!
- Take a few minutes to prepare before your practice. It is difficult to walk into the house after a day of work and traffic, and then say, "Okay, it's time to sit and meditate." It will not happen. Do something to calm and quiet your mind. Some examples are: listening to music, lighting incense or a candle, or walking.
- Set a realistic amount of time if this is a new practice. It is fine to begin with two to three minutes and slowly increase the time until you reach your target. Your goal might be five minutes per day and that will be quite effective.
- Leave your watch and cell phone in another room, because you will keep peeking. If time is a concern, use a timer with a soft alarm.

Remember, the most important aspect is to make your goals realistic and consistent. Keep your focus on progressing *one day at a time*. Your discipline and perseverance will pay off. Before you know it, you will be reading this week's entry again next year, having achieved success. Congratulate yourself, because you did it!

WEEK THREE

CHANGE

It is mid-January and we have set some goals for the upcoming year. Our calendars are already filled with all sorts of plans and many of them create new beginnings; however, there is one significant element that we seem to overlook: feelings. The familiar feelings of stress and anxiety crop up when we least expect them, even during happy times. In fact, they can accompany all of our other emotions and distract us from fully experiencing what is in front of us.

The following quote by Leo Buscaglia sheds light on this concept: "Change is life. Without change there would be no growth, no understanding, no relating, and no surprises. We are by nature changing beings. Still we seem to fear and resist it more than any other aspect of life."

I just got off the phone with my sister after wishing her a happy sixtieth birthday. She was not happy with the change (as well the publishing of her age); yet aging is part of the natural cycle of life. We age. Things change.

I remember how sad I felt when my daughters went off to college. My younger daughter recently graduated and moved back in and I began to wonder why I had been so sad! She will be leaving again soon and, again, I have a range of feelings.

We undergo many changes: graduations, weddings, anniversaries, new jobs, divorces, deaths, illnesses, and more. Each phase of life-change brings growth, discomfort, and opportunity. Yet, we resist these changes because we are creatures of habit. We are comfortable with how things are. We want our children to stay adorable, looking up to us like we are perfect in every way. (Oops, my mistake—this is not a fantasy book!)

So it is with every aspect of living, not only the big events. There will always be an ending and a new beginning, and every change impacts everyone involved. Since nothing stays stagnant and we should not get too attached to anything. But we do; we continue to resist the changes and when we finally let go we leave claw marks behind. No matter how tightly we hold on, change is guaranteed.

Many situations in life do not go as planned, and the struggle is painful. When the familiar ends and the new has not yet emerged, we are in the hallway in between, and it is not comfortable. At times it feels as if we will remain there forever.

Our minds' reaction to this discomfort wreaks havoc on our physical and emotional state. We see no end in sight because we have convinced ourselves that it will never change. But in the course of life, change happens, both positive and negative.

At some time or another every graduate seems to receive a popular Dr. Seuss book, *Oh, The Places You'll Go!* While looking around my home for the book, I noticed that I have two copies, one for each child. They are still in my house, even though both kids have graduated. (Hmmm, maybe it did not impress them the way it did me; or, maybe they knew this without Dr. Seuss telling them!)

The story begins with affirming how successful and wonderful the path will be. As the book progresses, there are many ups and downs to be endured, but in the end it all passes—both the easy times and the challenging times. An excerpt relates this point well:

> And when you're alone, there's a very good chance
> you'll meet things that scare you
> right out of your pants.
> There are some, down the road
> between hither and yon,
> that can scare you so much
> you won't want to go on . . . .

When things are going well, we want life to remain as it is. When things aren't going well, we want them to shift. Just like in Dr. Seuss' classic story, the path is filled with constant changes and it is helpful to remember that even the good things will ebb and flow.

Each moment brings change; as the moment passes a new moment emerges. Each and every breath is a new breath. Everything has a beginning, a crest, and an end—emotions, thoughts, sensations, events, breaths, and life itself. All of these things are constantly changing in a wavelike movement. We tend to focus on the most intense part and often get stuck there. When you look at an ocean wave, it begins with a calm assent and slowly climbs until it crests, then loses momentum and disappears. We will explore this significant concept throughout the book.

We have the ability to observe this wavelike movement when our attention is in the present moment. This will reduce our judgment about whether what is happening is good or bad, right or wrong—it is simply a moment-to-moment experience. Observing the waves of change inherent in life is an exquisite process and to resist it might keep you from seeing new opportunities.

Let's begin to cultivate the awareness of the changes within the wave with something simple, such as transportation.

- Focus on the movement of your car, bicycle, bus, subway, skates, boat, or any other vehicle you are in. Each movement begins, accelerates, slows, and stops. Notice the wavelike motion contained in the entire process.
- As you practice, notice if your mind is drifting away from what is happening. If so, become aware of your thoughts and bring your attention back to the moment-to-moment movement.
- This is an invitation to begin to cultivate the concept of a wave. Have fun with this exploration and keep an open mind.

The constant nature of change can offer us comfort because it represents something certain in life. When you really digest this fact, you will have an easier time rolling with the ups and downs inherent in your day. Whether it is traffic, a hot flash, a celebration, an illness, or loss, you can count on this simple phrase: *This too shall pass* . . . I guarantee you, it will.

WEEK 4

MOTIVATION FOR CHANGE: GARY'S STORY

I often think about what propels us into making changes. I have never heard anyone say—"My life is working well and I am exceedingly happy. I think it is time to make myself uncomfortable and do something to help me grow." No, what happens is that when we are in pain (the best motivator I know) that is what propels us to make adjustments to the way we function in life. We do not push ourselves out of our comfort zone unless we are up against the wall.

We already addressed the fact that change is constant—it is what we choose to do with it that makes the difference. Staying secure in the familiar can keep us stuck in old behaviors and habits. When we do this, we cut ourselves off from discovering our full potential.

The story I introduce is from a physician I have known for 25 years. We have both gone through many new beginnings, some wonderful and some painful. When I see him we laugh about how we handled situations so differently back then, before our lives changed.

Here is Gary's story:

> Let me start out by dispelling a myth that a lot of us from my generation have been taught as children. (I am 63 years old, and my parents were born right after the Depression.) The untruth is that if you live *right* and follow all the rules, your life will be perfect. *Wrong*.
>
> Fast forward to me as an adult, having a thriving medical practice, two children of my own and a beautiful wife, living comfortably in suburbia. My oldest

child was 14 and my youngest was 13. My baby was a violin protégé, extremely handsome, athletic, and too bright. We were so proud and arrogant and so judgmental. We were sure that if we coached the sports teams, went to all the teacher conferences, and all sat down together for dinner, we deserved these high-functioning, good looking children. Remember, we did follow all the rules.

To make a very long story short, our youngest became involved in drugs and alcohol. All the team captain positions went by the wayside. We were asked to withdraw our child from a very prestigious private school before they issued an expulsion. My life and the lives of everyone in our immediate family were spinning out of control. The more I tried to get everyone on track and come up with more punishment and/or rewards to reverse our son's behavior, the more the situation escalated. Finally, I was so depressed and anxious I went to see a psychiatrist. Perhaps a little green pill for anxiety could help me steward my family back on course. Why was this happening? We as parents did what we were supposed to do. These situations only happen to parents who are uninvolved, we thought. *Wrong.*

Throughout all this I didn't realize what a toll my attempts to handle the situation were taking on me and my family. Finally my psychiatrist convinced me, six sessions later, that I couldn't change my child's behavior. His advice was to step back and try to help myself, which might send a message to my troubled teen. "But doctor, how do I do that?" "Get a hobby or activity that is tailored just for you," he said. "If you are going to help your family, you need to recharge your batteries."

Allow me to interject that I always loved art, and had previously taken pottery and water color painting classes, but never finished the courses since I didn't excel. Soaring is very important to me. Anyway, the only class available was in acrylic painting. I halfheartedly signed up. I would not get any more of that green anxiety medicine from my psychiatrist if I didn't go. The classes seemed to be helping me so I wanted to continue. I knew a lot about art from my prior attempts taking classes, and I didn't realize that I could pull so much knowledge from my own collection and all the museums my wife and I had visited. Most importantly, my great teacher, Phil Carpenter, guided me in my "new" pursuit. He knew right out of the gate I had some talent and encouraged me to paint. And paint I did. It became a release and an energizer for me at the same time. I no longer wanted or needed those little green pills.

Thirteen years later (and painting almost every day) I am so blessed. My work is in four galleries throughout the Southeast; I frequently sell out my solo shows. In 2011, the art museum in Huntsville, Alabama, named me "Southeast Painter of the Year" and hung a solo exhibition for me.

My painting has shown me the power of tapping into a different part of one's self. It was the beginning of a whole new chapter of my life. While I still love practicing medicine, expressing myself through painting gives me the balance I need on a daily basis.

By the way, my child has reinvented himself. With our help and some other guidance, he has tapped into another side of himself. He graduated from college and received three job offers. To top it off, he just got married to a wonderful girl. Life doesn't have to be perfect, just well-lived, and each of us has the ability to go within to help deal with the imperfections.

As an obstetrician, Gary's job requires him to be responsible for new lives, which is stressful to say the least. I asked him how he deals with this, and he told me that painting is his outlet. His path was carved out by an unwelcome change, yet it propelled him in a new direction that fulfills him in a way that he never could have imagined.

This reminds me of a quote by Robert L. Stevenson: "To be where we are and to become what we are capable of becoming is the only end in life."

FEBRUARY

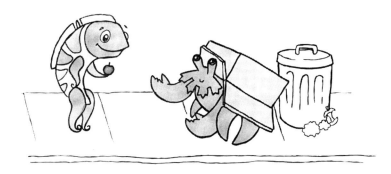

Love & Kindness

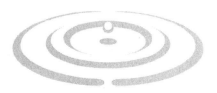

CUSTOM CALM

WEEK FIVE

COMPASSION

It was a beautiful day for a walk, so off my dog and I went to stroll through my neighborhood. As we approached a house, I watched an agitated family arguing in the driveway. By the time we had gone by, the father was yelling and telling his wife and small children to "shut up."

My immediate reaction was one of judgment and anger at the inappropriate behavior of the father. I wondered what caused his yelling and frustration. Unfortunately, this behavior happens in many relationships and most of the time, the person who is acting inappropriately really cares about the person he or she is hurting. I don't think any one of us is innocent of causing harm to another.

All traditions address this issue. It is right there in the Ten Commandments, so it must be of value! Rest assured, I am not an expert in the commandments, so I will use a simple teaching from yoga. It is the principle of non-violence.

Ahimsa is a word used in the yoga tradition, and it means non-violence or non-harmfulness in thought and action. Even though many of us try hard to be kind to others, somehow our harmful reactions still seep out. If we care about people in our lives, why would we want to cause them harm? It ends up creating pain for everyone involved, including ourselves.

This is a key point that needs to be explored. If we are harmful to ourselves in thought and action, no matter how hard we try not to, we will treat others in the same way. We touched on this in January when we focused on the need to show devotion and kindness to ourselves regarding things we are trying to accomplish. Let's take it a step further.

I remember an incident when I first began writing blog articles. Spelling is not my strong suit so I relied on spell-check. Spell-check is not infallible (however, it just corrected my lack of a hyphen in the word spell-check) but it missed an error I made. This resulted in the insertion of the alternate spelling, which changed the meaning of what I meant to say. I was grateful that a reader caught this and sent me a message correcting my error, but the way it was communicated was sarcastic and rude.

I wonder why the individual felt it necessary to correct me in a rude way. Even if I had given him the benefit of the doubt and assumed he was joking, it was still uncalled for. It would have been much more helpful if the message had been short, sweet, and to the point. Usually when a person is sarcastic and rude with others they treat themselves the same way.

Mistakes happen to us all. It is an opportunity to learn and grow. It is important to treat ourselves and others with compassion rather than getting stuck in the downward spiral produced by harmful comments.

We are much more receptive when input is communicated in a positive, solution-based manner. Practicing compassion when you or someone else makes a mistake will go a long way. Compassion can be thought of as a deep awareness of the suffering of another coupled with the desire to relieve it.

The Dalai Lama says: "Compassion is not religious business, it is human business, it is not luxury, it is essential for our own peace and mental stability, it is essential for human survival."

This quote from the Dalai Lama is compelling and accurate. Today, there is much focus on the pain caused by bullying and prejudice, making it even more apparent that change is needed now. Lack of compassion and awareness of the suffering of others is at the root.

The practice of compassion involves transforming our judgments and separateness toward others (even those we do not like) to becoming sensitive to their struggles and suffering. Your behavior affects the wellbeing of those around you, including yourself. The simple act of treating yourself and others with compassion is not about fixing anything or forgiving anyone, but showing up to life with openness, kindness, fullness, and peace.

Be aware that even a less significant situation, such as my spell-check error, can cause harm. A sarcastic comment did not cause me to suffer, but it was unkind and unnecessary. If we do not practice kindness on the small incidents, then what happens when we are faced with issues that really challenge us?

To begin cultivating compassion, we first need to become aware of *ahimsa* in thought and action. Let's take stock of how you treat yourself and others.

Ask yourself:

- How many times have I made a mistake and berated myself in the past few days? (It does not have to be an open affront, but calling yourself names like "stupid" or "idiot" is still harmful.)
- How often do I deny myself time to rest or play? (If you were tired and not feeling well, did you take a few minutes—at the very least—to relax and unwind?)
- How many times in the past few days did I have disparaging thoughts about others? (It still affects your peace and serenity even if you did not say a word.)
- How many times did I make a comment to someone else that was hurtful?

I am not asking you to do this to make you feel bad about yourself, but to help you see that even though you are a good, kind person, you are still human and there are times when you are unaware of how your actions influence yourself and others. Once you begin to notice your behavior and become conscious of its ripple effect, then you will have a choice to practice non-harmfulness. That will open the door for a life filled with compassion.

Remember what the Dalai Lama said about compassion: "Compassion . . . is essential for our own peace and mental stability." Your agitation and frustration will be replaced by kindness, compassion, ease, and joy.

How can you treat yourself and others with kindness today?

WEEK SIX

THE ULTIMATE VALENTINE'S GIFT

I was pleased to pick up the *New York Times* bestseller, *Love Is The Killer App: How To Win Business and Influence People.* It is a book for businesses, written by Tim Sanders. His emphasis is on bringing love and compassion to the workplace to foster success. I agree with Mr. Sanders' contention that compassion will not only foster success in business but throughout all areas of life.

The month of February specifically targets the idea of love as we are barraged with Valentine's Day cards, flowers, commercials, chocolate, special restaurant menus, and clothing. I am not so sure if the intention of these barrages is love, but the extra sales volume will propel the merchants to have smiles on their faces all day! Whatever the reason, the message is important and vital for a healthy state of mind.

Throughout our day, we have times when we are happy and centered, feeling compassionate, and filled with joy. At other times, as we explored in Week Five, we are faced with challenges, and our tendency is to shut ourselves off and become separate from those around us. We do not need to utter one word for negativity to ooze out from every cell. When we do this we perpetuate negativity, affecting those with whom we come in contact.

I was at a luncheon with friends, feeling quite happy and peaceful. A few of them were complaining about a problematic situation and the conversation became quite gloomy. Before I knew it, I could feel myself being pulled out of my peaceful mood. I was slimed—like in the movie *Ghostbusters*. Their negativity spewed all over the room! It took a lot for me not to take it on.

I have also been around people who exude happiness and joy. Their presence in a room is uplifting to those around them, including me! Joy is contagious, and so are the other moods.

We have all had times when we have stayed a bit too long stewing in the "woe is me" attitude, finding it comforting in some odd way. It is okay to visit that place from time to time, but we don't want to stay in the sludge too long; it will become like quicksand and can swallow us up before you know it. Even if we are not feeling loving or happy, we can choose how long we want to stay miserable.

There are simple ways to crawl out of the muck. Keep in mind that showing love can be a decision, rather than a feeling. Just a smile, a kind word, or a simple greeting to another can bring an upwelling of loving feelings in yourself, as well as in the other person. This simple action is a great beginning towards shifting your attitude and outlook upon life.

To begin to embody the changes from the inside-out, cultivate lovingkindness. I'm talking about a practice and a catalyst for change. In the Buddhist tradition, it is referred to as *metta*, meaning *friend* and *gentle*, and the practice will foster both.

Our feelings toward ourselves and others have an impact on our state of mind and how we perceive and react to the world around us. We find it easy to show lovingkindness for those we deeply care about. But what happens when a loved one is struggling? How do we get relief from worry and fear when there is nothing we can do? What about our more difficult relationships? How can we live amicably so we can remain or become calm and centered? These are lifelong challenges.

Whatever the situation, lovingkindness is the antidote for all relationships, good or bad. Can you begin with showing lovingkindness to yourself? This practice needs to begin with yourself, which for many of us is quite difficult.

Lovingkindness is a meditation, but do not fear; you do not have to sit on the mountaintop in Lotus position! This meditation is a tool to help you develop a loving state of being. It is a way to open up to receive and offer love, kindness, and compassion to others.

It might help to remember it is not a practice of forgiveness, but an acknowledgement that each one of us, even those whom we do not like, has the same desire for happiness. Some might not show it appropriately, but we are all human and connected in some way.

A valuable tool to foster lovingkindness consists of repeating a series of simple phrases with as much awareness as possible. There are many phrases that can be used. *The key is that you begin with yourself.* It is hard to wish for others what you do not want for yourself.

Here are some phrases with which you can begin:

> *May I (he, she or they) be happy.*
> *May I (he, she or they) know peace.*
> *May I (he, she or they) be safe and protected from inner and outer harm.*
> *May I (he, she or they) be free from suffering.*

- Repeat these phrases, beginning with "I" and then extend out to those you love. That might be plenty for a while.
- Then, add those about whom you feel neutral, such as the store clerk who is helping you.
- When you feel ready, add someone who is a challenge in your life. It could be someone you know personally, or someone you dislike. For example, it might be a politician.
- Then add someone who has harmed you or someone dear to you.

The practice of lovingkindness is simple and life changing. The intention of this practice is to help you live a life of joy and ease in all of your relationships. Imagine a life where you wake up each morning feeling a depth of connection with your own heart. That is the essence of Valentine's Day and it can last a lifetime. Try the practice for a few minutes each day and over time you will notice the changes. You might find that those around you seem kinder as well. It is the gift that keeps on giving.

WEEK SEVEN

WE ARE ALL DIVINE

As we continue to look at love, one piece that needs further investigation is being "a part of," rather than "apart from." As human beings, we tend to feel more at ease and relate to those with whom we identify. We like to be part of a herd— a group of animals of the same species sharing a specific purpose, and similar behaviors.

No, I am not comparing you to an animal; yet the fact is, we are mammals so we do have something in common. Our nature is to relate to others in our comfort zone, to travel as a pack. Your herd might be family, friends, business associates, fellow book club members, classmates, and many other relationships. Even though you spend time with them, many of these associations are based on mutual interest. Our interactions can be limited to common ground. There is connection, but it only takes us so far because it is based more on what we do rather than who we are.

You might be thinking, "First she calls me an animal and now she says my relationships are superficial?" I assure you, this is not a personal affront but a realistic view of our human condition. No matter how evolved we are, we still need some help breaking down the walls of separateness from others. This goes beyond our comfortable way of relating to one another.

Take a look at the term often used at the end of yoga classes: *Namaste*. It means, "I acknowledge and bow to the divine within you." The saying expands further: "When you are in that place in you and I am in that place in me, we are one." The word is used in India to greet one another. It does not matter whether it is a friend or stranger; they are treated in the same manner. *Namaste* includes you as well. Acknowledging first the divine in yourself and then to see it in others is a powerful practice.

When I teach yoga and movement, new students might find this greeting strange, but once they understand its meaning, they choose to say it. I remember having a student who for the longest time thought I was saying, "Have a nice day." When you think about it, acknowledging another and experiencing human connection will guarantee a nice day! In his book *Heal Thy Self*, Saki Santorelli, director of the Stress Reduction Clinic at University of Massachusetts Memorial Medical Center, comments on this greeting: "I believe that the active remembrance of this reality is crucial to our lives, our work, and our well-being." He says: "Our willingness to relate with another in this way is fundamentally healing."

In our culture, we connect only through the intellect, under some circumstances, such as in a work environment. However, living this way limits the possibilities of really knowing each other. The practice of relating through honoring the divine in one another is satisfying and uplifting. It opens our hearts and softens us in a way that touches those around us.

If you are concerned about softening and losing your tough, strong persona, fear not; you will be even more of a powerhouse than you are already! When you can see that we are all connected, you will access the inner stability that supports and sustains you in all situations. You will be able to see that you are part of something much greater than you. It is liberating when you do not recoil from another, no matter how uncomfortable you feel, because you acknowledge that they too, are divine.

Rest assured, I am not advocating that we all hold hands, sit in a circle, and sing *Kumbaya*. I also do not think it wise that you go up to a family member, boss, or stranger on the street, and say Namaste. (It would be entertaining to watch their reactions, but could put you at risk for clinical observation!) I also want to impart that this term and concept is not some "out there" notion of living.

It is much more than that. Begin to cultivate seeing beyond the external presence of others so you can appreciate them as another human being—divine, and no different from yourself. Even if you are an open-minded person who is generous and kind, you will still find this a bit challenging.

My experience with this reality was memorable. My husband and I accompanied a group to a homeless shelter in a rather rough part of town. It was Christmas time and we had filled backpacks with treats to distribute. This seemed like a generous and meaningful gesture but what struck me was the following occurrence: as the line was forming, we were told that after each person received his or her gift, we were to look them in the eye, shake their hand, and acknowledge them in some way. I must be honest, while this was out of our comfort zones, we felt tremendous gratitude and compassion. We greeted elders, teens, women, and men, with the recognition that deep down they were no different from us. It made a significant impression on both of us, developing our understanding of the possibilities for connection that we had not recognized before.

Try this for the next week:

- When you are in the presence of someone you already care about, look beyond your relationship with them and see the divine within them.
- When you are interacting with a stranger, be present with them and see if you can see beyond who you think they are and look for the divine within them.
- This one is the most challenging: The next time you pass someone that you find distasteful and want to avoid, understand that they, too, are human. If your first reaction is to turn away, look at them instead and acknowledge them in some way.

Whether it is a club member, business associate, classmate, friend, family, a disabled individual, or a homeless person, you will begin to see that we are all connected. You will become comfortable in any *herd* because you are stable and centered. Every day there will be new opportunities to deepen your connection to yourself and those around you.

Namaste.

WEEK EIGHT

HEART HEALTH

This month's theme of heart would not be complete without delving into one more area: keeping your heart healthy and fit. There is more to a healthy heart than diet and exercise. It involves that elusive, ever-popular word—stress. Yes, stress is capable of causing serious consequences and we will spotlight two areas that are linked:
1. Our physical heart health.
2. Our relationships with those around us.

I *Googled* the phrase "stress and heart disease" and got a staggering 30,700,000 results! Even the skeptic cannot negate that there is a relationship between the two. I am not an attorney (talk about stressful profession!), but in a court of law that number would serve as concrete evidence that, without a doubt, popular opinion is that stress and heart disease are linked.

There is a term that we are familiar with: fight-or-flight response. When we are in fight-or-flight response our entire body is affected. Some of the problems that arise are: increased heart rate and blood pressure, quicker breath rate, palpitations, and change in blood flow, all of which are negatively impacting your heart. Don't get me wrong, we need the fight-or-flight response. If we are being followed in a dark alley or if we see a child running into traffic we get the adrenaline rush needed to access tremendous strength and power. This can save lives. The problem arises when we respond in the same way when we break a nail (I am not minimizing the importance of a good manicure) or when our dog relieves himself on our carpet (frustrating, yes; life threatening, no).

Anxiety and stress stimulate the fight-or-flight response. Living our lives in fight-or-flight mode, we tend to stress over everything, and it wreaks havoc on our heart and relationships. With our February focus on love and heart, I found myself curious about why the heart is the symbol of love, since the human heart looks nothing like the heart on the Valentine card. I looked it up and found many theories, none of which made any sense. My husband will be happy about this finding because he feels it is a holiday made up by retailers—ever the romantic!

Even with this inconclusive finding, I will continue to explore how stress impacts our heartfelt relationships. We have seen how the heart can be strained by stress, but that is not the only problem that emerges. Think about a time when you were stressed out—I am sure you have many choices, but only pick one. The same warm, caring person who was cultivating lovingkindness has turned into a raving maniac. The cause? Stress. The Righteous Brothers sang about the consequences of stress in their popular hit, *You've Lost That Lovin' Feeling*.

When we look at our adoring children, partner, or friend, suddenly they do not look so wonderful. The love that we felt is replaced by our filter, which is distorted by stress. This has disastrous results. Now our feeling is separation, anger, or frustration—or all of the above. Our response to stress has robbed us of our inner capacity for love and care. We have drifted away from the space of Namaste that we looked at in Week Seven.

I know I have not painted a pretty picture and certainly do not want to stress you out, because that would be counterproductive. You are human and stress is part of life. You will find in future chapters I highlight stress because its impact is significant.

The good news is that there are many practices that will help. Because this month's focus is heart, I will direct the practice on helping you lower your stress response and level out your heart rate so you can once again find that loving feeling. One simple practice produces two benefits—now that's a deal!

When you are stressed, you tighten every muscle in your body; and since your heart is a muscle, it is affected, too. You cannot think your way to slowing down your heart rate, so you need to address your entire body. The tool that is always accessible is your breath.

When you are stressed, it is impossible to simultaneously stay tense and take a deep breath. Give it a try right now. Think about something that really bothers you and allow your body to react as it usually does. Now try to take a slow deep breath while staying tense. It will not happen.

The following basic breath awareness will help bring you back to the moment, averting the flight-or-flight response. Do not be fooled by the simplicity of the technique; it is very effective. It is the life preserver you can hang onto when you are drowning in anxiety.

- Sit comfortably with your spine upright on the floor or a chair.
- Uncross your arms and legs and feel your feet on the floor.
- Close your eyes or have a soft gaze.
- Begin to inhale and exhale through your nose. If this is problematic, breathe through your mouth.
- Bring your awareness to your breath without trying to influence it in any way. Simply follow it with your mind.
- Notice the quality of your breath.
- Notice the depth, pace, and rhythm.
- Find the place where the breath feels the most evident and focus your attention there—it might be your heart center, your rib cage, or belly.
- Take a few more easy breaths and notice how you feel.

This week, practice the above technique so you can experience the immediate calming benefits of focused breathing. Get in the habit of taking a few slow, easy breaths at the onset of a small frustration (there will be many opportunities), and you will begin to catch yourself before you get to full fight-or-flight reaction. Remember, even something as simple as breathing takes time to learn, so be patient. It's good for you, and your heart will thank you.

MARCH

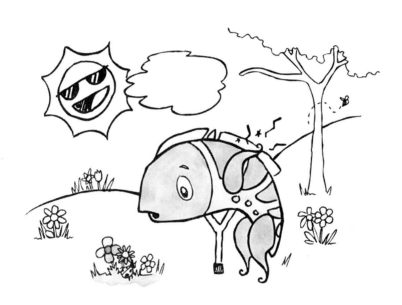

Pain & Illness

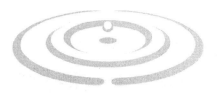

C U S T O M C A L M

WEEK NINE

AWARENESS

This month as we focus on pain and illness, let's first take a look at injuries that could have been easily avoided. We stub our toe, trip, pull something, fall, or more seriously, we crash into something. The one thing that most accidents have in common is that we were not giving our full attention to what we were doing.

This brings to mind a recent incident. My older daughter was riding her bicycle in the appropriate bike lane in Chicago. Someone parked on the side of the street and opened his door without paying attention. Her bicycle went one way and she the other. The fall separated her shoulder. This is an example of an accident that could have been easily avoided. The driver was on auto pilot and not looking at his surroundings. (Yes, he got a ticket; yes, he has insurance—no worries.)

Awareness can be thought of as the ability to perceive, feel, or to be conscious of events, situations, and/or objects. The reality is, we have the ability but we do not fully use it.

In this case, the individual who caused the accident was not in the state of mind where he was conscious of the oncoming bicycle. This behavior is familiar to many of us. We might say we are distracted, unaware, zoned out, or in a fog. There are medical reasons that can cause a foggy mind, but for most of us, we simply do not pay attention.

Jon Kabat-Zinn wrote a popular book called *Wherever You Go, There You Are*. The truth is that we are more in tune with the Beatles' song—*Here, There, and Everywhere*. We often are not where our feet are planted, which is the cause of many accidents. Sometimes it takes an injury to realize that had we been more present in our actions, we probably could have avoided the accident. There are many examples of this, as demonstrated in the following recent Atlanta Journal Constitution article titled, *In yoga class, play it safe:*

> A student was injured in a yoga class as he was pushing himself to go deeper into a pose. He wanted to go further because he was watching others in the class (or maybe he wanted to try out for Cirque du Soleil). Whatever the reason, he realized after his knee snapped that he had pushed his body too far. The problem arose from not paying attention to what his body was telling him. After his injury he shifted his focus to a practice that was mindful and more internal, where he checked in with his body.

Unfortunately, it often takes physical pain to remind some of us that we have a body, something we often take for granted. We are reminded that we need to take better care of ourselves. I will take this opportunity to say that yoga is not a contortion act, but an internal experience of exploration using breath and movement, so anyone is able to do it. We just need to give it our full attention to avoid overdoing it.

Henry Miller once said, "Our own physical body possesses a wisdom which we who inhabit the body lack. We give it orders which make no sense." Yes, our body has infinite wisdom. When we partake in any physical practice, whether sports, weight-training, walking, yoga, Pilates, dance, or anything else, the key is to stay aware of the information coming from your body. Looking back at the explanation of awareness, think, "Am I able to perceive, to feel what I am participating in, or am I doing it mechanically with my mind somewhere else?"

I find that our bodies tell us the truth and our minds judge. We allow our minds to take charge and negate the body's wisdom. Both need to be heeded. This way you can be aware of your thoughts, while adapting your activity to meet the needs of your body. You will be effectively working with your body, not against it. Your body will thank you.

Back in my youth I used an exercise video and the theme was to "make it burn." Today that premise still holds and is referred to as: "No pain, no gain." I had a client who lived with that motto until her body imploded with chronic illness. I watched her struggle with letting go of her forceful attitude and need to feel a big stretch, to adopting a softer, more compassionate way of practicing. She received many physical and emotional benefits from her new approach and it served her well. It is challenging for her, but she can tell the difference in her health when she is overdoing, rather than listening to, her body.

There is value in challenging yourself and setting goals, as we discovered during January, but keep in mind the point made by Henry Miller: it needs to make sense. It does not make sense to over-do and abuse your body. All activity is an opportunity to practice being aware of yourself and your surroundings, while participating fully.

At times, my students and clients need some reassurance to know if they are pushing too much. I answer them with a bit of humor as I say: "I am okay with your discomfort, but not with your pain."

How do you discern if you are pushing too much or if you are really able to go a bit further? These following simple tips will help:

- If you are in pain, back off.
- If you are comparing yourself to someone else, chances are you are overdoing it.
- If you are going further because a teacher told you to, make sure to check in with your body.
- If you feel a stretch and you cannot breathe into it, you need to ease out a bit.
- If you are holding your breath to be able to maintain the pose or stretch, then back out. You must be able to breathe when exercising.
- It is okay to push your body, but remember to listen to what it needs.

A great way to begin cultivating awareness is when you are participating in physical activity. Notice what your mind is telling you and check in with your body. Stay present with your actions, even if they are things you do every day. This way, you can be where your feet are planted rather than stumbling over them!

WEEK TEN

ACCEPTANCE

Out of all of the definitions of acceptance, this is my favorite: "Acceptance is being willing to have the experience you are already having versus struggling to escape your own experience."

Its origin intrigues me; the Yoga of Awareness professional training at Duke University Integrative Medicine. It is a principal consideration when dealing with challenging illnesses and chronic pain.

What is "integrative medicine" and why is it of such importance that leading universities are spending time and money on research and training in it? Let's go back to Hippocrates. He said: "It is more important to know what sort of person has a disease than to know what sort of disease a person has."

In a nutshell, Hippocrates just explained integrative medicine. We are more than our illness and the entire person must be included in healing. The days of "take two aspirins and call me in the morning" are over.

Integrative medicine is a whole-person approach designed to treat the individual, not just the disease. There is a partnership between the patient and the doctor where the goal is to treat the mind, body, and spirit, all at the same time. It is hardly "New Age" as it has been around since 460 BC, so I feel safe in saying it has withstood the test of time. Esther Sternberg, MD, from the National Institutes of Health, says, "Patients want to be considered whole human beings in the context of their world." Stress triggered by illness and pain result in serious consequences so these externalities must be addressed.

What does the definition of acceptance have to do with all this? Everything. When we experience illness or pain, it is natural to have feelings of wanting the pain or illness to change. The problem arises when our feelings propel us into judging what we are going through as unacceptable. This begins a spiral of negative thinking and when our minds react and tighten, so do our bodies. There is now a layer of tension that intensifies the existing sensation. Think about it; if you were able to stay present with your pain or illness and notice sensation from a more neutral mindset, without layering judgment, frustration, and anger, the experience would be different. It is the struggle and resistance to what is happening that adds more pain and stress to an already challenging situation.

Let me give you an example from my experience of applying this principle to pain and illness.

I developed shingles which affected my face; the sensation was quite intense, especially when I brushed my teeth. As I stood at the sink I could feel my body tighten up at the thought of the extreme sensation I was about to endure. I took a breath, felt my feet on the floor, and proceeded to brush my teeth. I made a decision to notice the discomfort without labeling it good or bad. The intense sensation did come but quickly passed as I stayed with it. The irony is that our resistance and wish to escape our reality exacerbates what is happening. The saying "what we resist, persists," is quite true. Another moral of this story is to carefully choose what you teach, because you will have many opportunities to make sure you know your material!

I learned the following concept years ago: "It is what it is, while it is, the way it is" and I have added one more line "until it changes." This understanding is quite freeing. The philosopher Renee Descartes proposed that there was a definite relationship between how we perceive a situation and how we experience it: when we react to what is, we intensify our experience.

While it might sound like I am asking for miracles, I promise it can be done. I know because I have seen my clients make the change from judgment to perception, and you can, too. I am not implying that we give up or resign to our situations. My point is that when you are able to bring your attention to the moment and you make the choice not to layer judgment upon it, you can feel calm and centered.

I admit that remaining in the moment when you are in pain seems to be a lofty concept. Pain and illness are not to be taken lightly. We have actual pain and then we layer our resistance and judgment upon our experience. Our resistance and judgment intensifies the pain. The good news is that we have control over our reaction to what is happening. There is much more happening in any given moment then the pain we feel. I will share a story from a client to clarify this concept.

Janice had undergone many treatments for cancer with complications that left her with many side effects. When she went for her mammogram, the pain was so intense that it brought her to tears. She asked me for some suggestions. I told her that as the mammogram was being administered, there was more happening in the moment. Because her sole focus was on the intense pain, the sensation was magnified. I suggested that while the mammogram was taking place, to also feel her feet on the floor, notice her breathing, notice what was in her line of sight, notice the pressure of the equipment, temperature, and so on. There was more happening in the moment than the pain. Janice later emailed me that she employed these techniques and reported that the procedure did not bring her to tears as it had in the past, and the pain was less intense. She said that noticing her feet on the floor and her breathing helped a lot. Although practicing presence in the moment is not the miracle cure to avoid discomfort, it is an effective process for helping yourself through challenging situations.

Next time you feel sensation, notice there is more happening in the moment. The sensation will still be there, as it is part of what is happening at the time, but engage your other senses as well. You will shift away from layering more tension onto the struggle to noticing what is happening as it is happening.

Remember: It is what it is, while it is, the way it is, until it changes. And it will change ... *That is guaranteed.*

WEEK ELEVEN

COMMUNITY

We can do it together. You are not alone. We can do what I cannot. These sayings carry a universal message: no matter what is happening in life or how badly you feel, you can find community for mutual support. Support groups are effective because a group of total strangers want to help one another.

As we continue to delve into pain and illness, I will refer back to the Week Six theme of love and kindness. It is a main ingredient in healing nurtured through community support. At times we are faced with difficult situations, leaving us feeling isolated and alone. It might be conflict, addiction, illness, or loss and those around us try to help, but they cannot give the appropriate support because they have not walked in our shoes.

A community where the group shares common ground provides great healing.

There are camps throughout the world that support children with serious illnesses, disabilities, and other challenges. Twin Lakes is one of those venues and Camp Twitch and Shout is for children with Tourette syndrome. Camp Sunshine helps those with cancer. Here are some comments from two of the children who attended those camps:

> I wake up every morning thinking that I'm one day closer to camp.

> The best thing about camp is Fun and Fitting In. I meet (sic) a real nice friend. She is the first very best friend I have ever had. Megan is my best friend because she understands. Camp Sunshine helped me feel like a regular kid, I did not have to worry about my scars on my tummy or on my chest and no one made fun of me. Every day was so fun. I can't wait until next summer.

What is significant for these children is the hope they feel while at camp. They see others, with the same struggles, from all walks of life and ages, just being kids and having fun. They are more than their circumstances, and their illnesses or conditions are certainly not the focus. The common ground shared at camp provides them with support and community that they could not have gotten from others.

I am fortunate to teach and design programs at The Cancer Support Community Atlanta, and what strikes me most is the care and love of the entire community. It does not matter if someone has cancer, had cancer, or supported or lost a loved one with cancer; what is evident is the mutual support the members give each other as they share their experiences, strengths, and hopes. Wealth, religion, ethnicity, age, gender, and size do not matter—the members of this community rally around one another.

The environment is upbeat and the focus is on enjoying life. What is so remarkable is that they do not try to fix one another. Instead, they listen and provide encouragement, always welcoming a new person. They understand, because they have lived it.

No matter how I am feeling when I walk in, my spirits are lifted. I take great pleasure in watching students unwind, enjoy the moment, and learn how to take care of themselves. I always leave feeling calm, centered, and inspired. Every time I teach at The Cancer Community I am reminded that we are all connected.

This brings me to another important reason why these communities are so effective. Their emphasis is on the solution and supporting one another on how to live life on life's terms. They come together not only because they share common ground but also because they gain a new perspective as they learn through love and kindness that they are much more than their illness or situation.

Let's use an analogy to expand upon this important point.

Visualize yourself as an iceberg. The tip of the iceberg is all that can be seen above water and by the public. It is covered with your identities—who you think yourself to be: a parent, child, employee, employer, friend, teacher, athlete, Southerner, and so on.

Consider this: What happens when one of your identities changes? You were healthy and now you are ill, your child goes to college and now you have no one to nurture, you were fired from your job, or you move. Who are you now?

Remember that the span and depth of your iceberg is massive. The tip is only one ninth of what you see (I love the Internet; I feel so knowledgeable), and if you only focus on that small fraction, you will miss most of the iceberg. Now, take a look beneath the water's surface. What will you find there? It is important that you recognize that you are so much more than the identities that cover the tip of the iceberg.

When we are young it is easier to see past the top of the iceberg and know we are more, because children freely embrace what they are doing without feeling limited by externals. The child's description of camp illustrates this. The campers felt part of a community that recognized them for who they were as human beings, rather than labeled with their illnesses, handicaps, or conditions. They do not look at themselves in that way because their circumstances are not their identity, but only a small part of who they are.

As we get older it is easier to get caught up in our identities and when we do this, we limit ourselves. Your capacity is vast and you have an inner depth greater than you can imagine. You are more than your body and more than your mind. You are more than your illness, your pain, your circumstances. You are part of something greater, and when you are embraced by community and get the loving support you need, you will know in every fiber of your being that you really are more.

Who do consider yourself to be beyond the tip of the iceberg?

WEEK TWELVE

EMPOWERMENT

Pain is epidemic in the United States. According to the findings of the June 2011 study by the Institute of Medicine, *Relieving Pain in America,* chronic pain affects about 100 million American adults—more than those affected by heart disease, cancer, and diabetes combined. Pain also costs the nation up to $635 billion each year in medical treatment and lost productivity.

The *Associated Press* article by Lauran Neergaard, June 29, 2011 commented:

> All kinds of ailments can trigger lingering pain, from arthritis to cancer, spine problems to digestive disorders, injuries, to surgery. Chronic pain can also be a disease all its own.

Dr. Doris Cope, pain chief at University of Pittsburgh Medical Center states: "Too many think a pill's the answer, when there are many ways to address pain. The population is getting older and less fit, and more survivors of diseases such as cancer live for many years with side effects from treatments."

Another report entitled, *Military to Implement Integrative Medicine for Comprehensive Pain Management*, published by *The Bravewell Collaborative*, highlighted the issue of pain among military personnel.

> In June 2011, senior military medical leadership met with *The Bravewell Collaborative* and renowned scientists and physicians at the Pentagon to discuss improving pain management for warriors and veterans through the use of integrative medicine. Clinical research showed a reduction in pain scores by as much as 50 percent.

Now for some more positive news (always the optimist) about the situation: there are a multitude of methods that we can employ to help ourselves and they do not involve a drink or drug. (Yes, some consider me a killjoy.)

Earlier this month I referred to the identities beneath the iceberg and I will take that a step further. Chronic pain and illness can take over our lives and we can become attached to our situation, even though we really want it to improve.

I recently worked with a client who was struggling with chronic illness, pain, and anxiety. As I worked with him, I could see how my recommended simple, basic practices were helpful in addressing his issues. I invited him to practice a bit each day, modifying practices to meet his needs. We worked with activities that interested him most to cultivate a new perspective in viewing his situation and empowering change. During the last session I had with him, he was beginning to feel relief and was excited to make the next appointment. The next day he cancelled and I never heard from him again. Why?

I see this happen with chronic illness. His illness had become his identity and he became attached to his situation. It also gave him a few perks. He was treated with kid gloves with positive attention from others as they were concerned about his well-being. He had become lost in his illness and was stuck in the spiral; he actually resisted feeling better.

I understand how easily this can happen. After the birth of my second child, I developed Lupus, a chronic illness. It could have derailed me from everything I used to enjoy but I consider myself lucky to have had tools to support me in living and embracing all of who I am. The same practices I am recommending sustained and empowered me and today I do not consider that I have Lupus at all. I have been symptom-free for many years.

Here are some techniques that address two common health issues:

Chronic Pain and Illness

One of the most effective practices for chronic pain is deep body relaxation. We do not realize how much tension we hold within our bodies. When we learn to systematically soften and let go, we both relax our bodies and diffuse our focus on the areas of discomfort.

Here is a very basic body scan to guide you through this process. Throughout this practice, direct the breath into each area of your body while noticing sensations or emotions, pleasant or unpleasant:

- Bring awareness to your mouth and notice your entire mouth.
- Notice through your ears, around to your eyes and nose.
- Become aware of your entire skull.
- Notice your neck, shoulders, down your arms—both front and back, right into your fingertips, and then back up again.
- Become aware of your throat.
- Continue to notice down your torso, through your entire chest as you breathe and soften.
- Span your awareness around your sides and notice your entire back, including your shoulder blades, ribs, waist, and down through both hips.
- Now, notice your entire torso, front, back, and throughout the core.
- Draw your attention down your legs, front, and back, right through to your toes, and then back up again.
- Allow your awareness to rest in your pelvic bowl, breathing and softening.
- Now, feel your body as a whole and rest in the awareness of your entire body.

When you slowly scan your body in this way, it is important to allow your breath to be relaxed and easy, staying in each area for a few breaths. Stay present, and if judgment or thoughts arise, compassionately notice them and draw your awareness back to your body. If a different order works better for you, feel free to make up your own.

Back and Neck Pain

Two common complaints I hear about are low back and neck pain (a show of hands please for those who do not have this issue!). The gentle stretching I employ decompresses both areas. Also, learning how to bend is important to protect your back.

Let's begin with some interesting facts about lumbar pressure that I found in *Rehabilitation of the Spine: A Practitioner's Manual*.

- Sitting hunched over a desk: 200 lbs.
- Sitting leaning back on chair with low back rounded: 150 lbs.
- Standing with leaning forward posture: 200 lbs.
- Standing in proper alignment: 100 lbs.
- Lying flat on back: 55 lbs.
- Lying flat on back with knees elevated: 25 lbs.

My editor often shows up to our meetings in high heels, which exacerbates her existing back pain. I assure her that she will still be a fabulous editor wearing flats (okay, a low heel with a sole that bends) that will reduce compression on her spine. She's beginning to notice the effect her shoes have on her body.

Throughout this book you will find different techniques to help relieve the strain on your spine, but here's a quick vocabulary lesson: The *lumbar* region of your spine is the main culprit and is located in the lowest portion, just above your sacrum. The *sacrum* is the heavy, flat triangular-shaped bone at the base of your spine. Your *sitting bones* are part of your pelvis, and these are the bones you feel when you sit.

I will highlight a few tips to relieve back pain:

- Think of your body as having angles and your joints as hinges.
- Become aware of your legs and press them firmly into the floor.
- Bend your knees.
- Hinge at your hips.
- Lengthen your sitting bones out behind you.
- Keep your sacrum flat and lengthened.
- Draw your abdominals in toward your spine. They are a thumb's length below your navel.

Practice these exercises in front of a mirror to make sure your sacrum stays flat and that you lead with your sitting bones. When you bend this way, you get the added benefit of strengthening your legs and abdominals. This is also a great way to come up and down from a chair, which we will look at later. Do this regularly and you'll notice less strain in your lumbar area.

Pain and illness will impact most of us in some way throughout our lives, but suffering is optional. We can help ourselves out of the vicious cycle of pain and illness and live a calm, peaceful, fulfilling life. It is within your grasp, so why not reach for it?

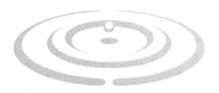

C U S T O M   C A L M

APRIL

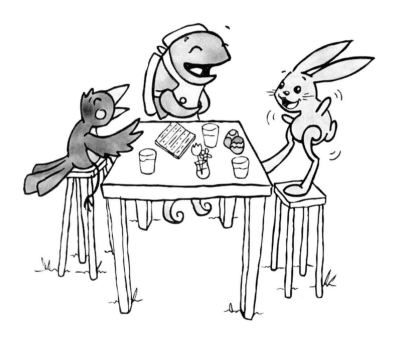

Emergence

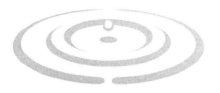

C U S T O M C A L M

WEEK THIRTEEN

LIGHTEN UP!

April Fools' Day marks the beginning of April and the spring season. I was curious about the holiday's origin and thought I would pass along what I found in my research.

It began in the 1500s in France with the change of New Year's Day from April 1 to January 1. With the slow communication in those days, many did not hear about the change until years later. Others refused to acknowledge the change, and those people were labeled fools. Thus began the tradition of prank playing on April 1st. Many countries celebrate this day as both the onset of spring and a reason to be playful.

Okay, so these facts are not life-changing, but they bring up an interesting question: Why do so many of us find it appealing to play a joke on someone? One reason is that it gives us the opportunity to lighten up and play because we take life so seriously and we need an excuse to get a bit silly. Let's take this a bit further.

Our lives are over-scheduled and busy, with pressure coming at us from many directions. This is much of what underlies the stress pervading our society. So we try a variety of activities in our efforts to chill out. In our quest to be healthy, we do some form of exercise—we work out, jog, dance or hike, to name a few. Perhaps we join a yoga class to help relieve stress, but in our rush to relax we get a speeding ticket. All of these activities are beneficial and can be enjoyable, but this is not the type of fun I am speaking about.

Because our lives are so full, we attempt to plan some fun time. Most often, we need to wait for some off time on the weekend or the long-awaited vacation. When we finally make it to our scheduled time off, we are too tired to really lighten up. Let's use golf as an example. We begin our game taking pleasure in the sunshine but as the day progresses, clubs are thrown, tempers are lost, and frustration mounts because of a poor shot, a slow group in front of us, or a missed putt (my personal favorite). When we finish the four or five hours of "play," we wonder why we are not refueled for the week to come. Then, when asked about the day, we report that we had a great time!

We do have those activities that leave us quite refreshed, but the Monday alarm goes off and we are off and running once again. Eventually, we get burnt out and stressed not remembering how to be fun-loving and spontaneous. This topic fits with the theme of emergence because as we take on more and more responsibilities we lose our spontaneity. You might be thinking, "Yes, Ellen, this is true but with so much on my plate, fun is a luxury I do not have. Maybe after the kids are grown and I retire." We wait and wait and fun takes a back seat.

Fun does not have to wait until vacation time, a class, a date, or a game. With requirements like that, even when we participate in these events, we often are unable to unwind enough to really be playful. How do we make this change when there are few opportunities for a break?

First, there needs to be a shift in attitude. We take ourselves and those around us very seriously and forget our sense of humor. You might remember the physician, Dr. Patch Adams. His research and outlook were based on the need for laughter, joy, and creativity as an integral part of the healing process.

There have been studies about the benefits of a smile, even one that is not authentic. A smile will increase dopamine levels (neurotransmitters affecting pleasure), helping to elevate your mood. I think this is why they are finding that Botox injections around the mouth improve one's mood. (Go figure!) If humor and laughter help those with physical and emotional problems, imagine how your life would improve if you laughed more, too!

Have you ever noticed the behavior of someone interacting with a baby? They seem to turn into a different person, making up words, making faces, smiling, and carrying on, doing anything to get the baby to react. I would venture to say that if they behaved this way without a baby present they would be carted off to someplace safe! Because acting silly toward an infant is socially acceptable, we give ourselves permission to let go.

It is easy to have fun with the simple things in life. I have a friend who works in a highly stressful job and we were getting pedicures. She had picked out a common color for her toes and I encouraged her to try something fun, like blue. She did this and then I suggested she have a flower painted on her big toe, and she hesitantly agreed. As she examined her toes, she got so excited at how much fun they were to look at that she decided to make this part of her future pedicures.

We need to lighten up throughout our day-to-day living. Many of our responsibilities are not fun and can be stressful. The attitude you bring to your tasks will make a significant difference. When your perspective is one of "having" to do a task, you set yourself up for drudgery. We can choose to bring humor into our day, even laughing at our own mistakes. Nothing we do is that earth-shattering (sorry to inform you overachievers) and if we laugh we will be more present in our lives.

Take time each day to be silly and playful. Sing, laugh, joke, and be light hearted without concern about how you look. Even if you are in a conservative company, try it. I do not know of anyone who has been fired for being upbeat, positive and friendly. As strange as this might sound, add this to your to-do list until it becomes natural.

Here is one assignment to get you started. I was inspired by a simple practice from Amy Weintraub, author of the book *Yoga Skills for Therapists*. It is a quick, effective mood lifter.

- Tuck your chin downward.
- Curl your lips in an upward direction.
- Slowly lift your head while keeping your lips curled upward.
- Yes, this is a smile.
- Now, go enjoy the day!

It can be done at any time and takes only a few seconds. If you are struggling to give yourself permission to try this, even in privacy, what do you think is getting in your way? I know this is not easy for many of us, which makes it that much more imperative. Remember, life is to be enjoyed not endured. You deserve to laugh and lighten up every day.

There was a popular television commercial with the slogan, *"Try it, you'll like it."* Yes, a smile, colorful pedicure, or simply whistling a tune will make a difference. You will be surprised by how refreshed you feel.

WEEK FOURTEEN

EASTER AND PASSOVER

The following quote by Joseph Campbell is a wonderful introduction to the spring season. He said, "We must be willing to get rid of the life we've planned; so as to have the life that is awaiting us . . . The old skin has to be shed before the new one is to come."

Passover and Easter have the theme of emergence. With winter behind us, we step outside to enjoy festivals, concerts, and other spring events. It is the season when we graduate high school or college, attend weddings, and plan visits to the waterfront anticipating the start of summer. All of these celebrations mark new phases of life, and, yes, we like any opportunity to express joy.

Spring offers us many opportunities to watch changes in nature. All around us there is new growth. Last year's leaves have died off and the flowers, plants, and trees are sprouting with an array of colors and fragrances. There is rebirth everywhere you look and it is absolutely beautiful.

If we study nature, we learn that there is a process that must take place, and sometimes it is difficult and uncomfortable. The budding of the new foliage looks lovely, but it brings with it some discomfort. In Atlanta, the blooming of azaleas, pine trees, and other foliage create a pollen count of more than 6,000, along with unpleasant allergies, eye irritations, and yellow cars.

Animals must also go through discomfort inherent in transformation. A butterfly must struggle to break out of its cocoon. If it is broken open too early, the butterfly will die. To make room for the emergence of the new, the old must first die off, and that can feel extremely uncomfortable.

Let's take it a step deeper as we explore the April holidays: Passover and Easter. These holidays include foods that represent certain aspects of the stories that are told (matzo ball soup and chocolate bunnies are worth celebrating on their own), but there is more to these holidays than celebrating and remembering what happened in the past.

The Passover story is about release from the bondage of slavery into freedom. Easter is a time of rebirth and renewal. Both embody the theme of transformation and new beginnings—a second chance at life.

We commonly think of bondage as being under the control or influence of something powerful. Passover marks the freedom of the Israelites from Egyptian bondage. In this case, the power that bound the Israelites was from other human beings. Today, we still live in bondage, but not from another person; it is self-imposed and stems from our mind. We are slaves to our own thoughts. We get trapped by our way of perceiving life and see no way out, stunting our capacity to grow and move in new directions.

The renewal and rebirth of Easter can also release us from bondage. There are times in life when we are stuck, bound by our circumstances and way of behaving. How liberating to know we can begin again at any time.

Our busy mind generates a fog over what we see, obscuring what is possible. It stems from historical and current thoughts and emotions that form our patterns and belief systems. When we become stuck in old beliefs, then everything we do and see is observed through the same old eyes. To see our situation with a new outlook reminds me of the newest evolution of televisions, crisp and clear. Life can be so much brighter and crisper when the fog lifts.

The renewal and rebirth of Easter and the freedom from bondage of Passover carry principles that we can integrate into our lives. The key principle is that we all have the innate capacity to live with inner peace and joy. It is a time to let go of old thoughts and belief systems in order to be receptive to something different.

One of the key concepts in Zen Buddhism is to see things with a beginner's mind, maintaining an attitude of openness and eagerness. Allow yourself to live with a beginner's mind, as if you are experiencing it all for the first time. Even if you do not have anything to take the place of your old beliefs, you can begin with a clean slate; this will allow space for the emergence of the new.

When you are open, life is more exciting and you experience everything at a much deeper level. The simple act of being willing to break old patterns will create space, and you will notice that things begin to change. It is a powerful and empowering practice—a true release from bondage followed by emergence. How do we begin to break old patterns? The first step is to be aware that they exist—you cannot change what you do not know about. Let's start with something small:

- Cultivate a mindset of being open and willing to change rather than using brute force. This is the first step to change, and just being open will prove quite effective. The process of simple awareness will jump-start the change.
- Think about one small behavior that you would like to change. Start with something easy. You might find that noticing your thoughts or speech will help you select something to work on. Choose one behavior you wish to change and begin to notice it. Soon it will become annoyingly obvious. When you see it happening, take a breath and feel the connection of your feet to the surface beneath you. This will help quiet your mind.
- Be kind and gentle with yourself, as it might not be comfortable to see what keeps you stuck. It is like the children's arcade game "whack-a-mole" where one mole pops up and you hit it with a hammer; then another pops up. This will happen with your chosen behavior, and then one day a new mole will pop up. That is great progress.

Don't forget: Rome was not built in a day, and neither were your old patterns and behaviors. The process of change and emergence is not always comfortable, so notice the small changes. It takes time. Be patient and kind to yourself with the process.

Renewal is a natural process as exemplified in Easter and Passover. When the shackles of your mind begin to fall away, freedom and clarity will take its place. It will bring new meaning to the holidays as you see the brilliance of spring through new eyes. Happy Spring!

WEEK FIFTEEN

EMERGENCE FROM WORKAHOLISM: SHELLIE'S STORY

Shellie's story poignantly illustrates the messages in Week Fourteen about Easter and Passover—letting go, emergence, and freedom. I am inspired by her honesty and journey.

It all began as an adventure—driven by the desire to succeed and the opportunity to influence and inspire others. It felt meaningful, purposeful, and, best of all, it allowed me to set out to work each day ready, willing, and able to change people's lives for the better. It seemed noble to help others reach goals, provide for my family, and to love what I do. Many dream of having such a rewarding career, so I took care of my employees, my family, my boss, and friends. Isn't that what we all want to do—be happy and make others happy too?

It turns out that being good at changing people's lives through my business resulted in nice bonus checks, trips around the world, audacious recognition, promotions, and notoriety. Red alert... being the recipient of all these things can change a person!

The last thing I remember clearly... I was on stage receiving the "you're the best in the whole world and we all love you and hate you for being so awesome at everything" award... camera's flashing, crowds cheering... then "fade out."

I believed that I could change lives, make lots of money, be a great mom, wife, boss, friend, employee... you get the idea... do it all! After a long run of doing just that I began to realize that something was missing.

I had no idea what. I just knew that all of these things were not making ME happy and all of the sudden, at 40, I realized that I was pretty important. Not the "I" that was successful and in the spotlight, admired by so many—"how do you do it all?" they would say— but the "i" that was hiding inside that woman who seemed to have it all and keep it all together.

I can't recall how the self-discovery evolved or that exact moment when I knew, but sometime early in my 40th year I realized I was not happy with ME (ME = I + i) and evidently my unhappiness had been my inner reality for quite some time. Many people who loved me, and some who didn't, knew it long before I did. I tend to be (ugh) stubborn, so the ones who loved me just kind of stepped back in fear as I began to unravel.

I began to realize that the catalyst to my undoing might just be my unconscious addiction to praise and success in that rock star job. I didn't take it too well. I was losing my edge! It sucked. The truth is, I was genuine and I was good at it until I became addicted to the success. WOW, what a revelation. But, it defined me! So I continued on . . . being miserable, getting sick, losing my edge, and being frightened to walk the halls at work thinking a saboteur was lurking just around the corner (because anyone who didn't like me was surely out to get me right?). My weekends became little more than rejuvenation to get on yet another plane Monday morning and do it over again. My family members stayed a safe distance back and friends listened with sympathy at my sad story of a miserable job. Asking me if I was OK could lead to disaster. Of course I was OK! I could handle it. The job, the boss, and the stress were not going to get the best of me. Denial. Avoidance. Insanity.

So one day before my 41st birthday . . . yes, I got fired! You know when you see something happening before it does but you just ignore it—hoping it won't happen or maybe you are just wrong? I was devastated. Not surprised, just devastated. I knew things were bad. I hated my job. I just never imagined that the decision might not be in my hands. So after a day of tears and feeling betrayed I celebrated my birthday and determined that this would be a turning point.

What I learned . . . turns out the saboteur wasn't around the corner after all. SHE was ME! Ouch! My identity was so dependent on my career that I had absolutely NO vision of myself outside of that. I was stunned! You know, like the boxer who gets the final blow but stays on his feet bobbing around the ring.

It took some time to convince myself that I had purpose and worth without that job. My friends were kind, supportive, and timid. Talking with me about "what happened" was about as dangerous as feeding wild game. There was always a chance that I would display some new emotion. It was always a gamble to bring it up. I couldn't even say I was fired—I would say, "when I left" or something benign that didn't imply my failure. Others continued to tell me how great I was and all the reasons I would bounce back and be better than ever, but before I could see what they saw I had to take some time to look in the mirror, dig deep, and figure out who the hell I am without the job, the title, and the positional power. I set out to figure out how life could go on after being fired!

First, I practiced sitting still without being productive. Then, I began to think about what was really going on? I made an amazing discovery . . . I had spent much of my life doing what I thought I was supposed to do. I now realized that have options! I am allowed to consider what I want! So next—what did I want? This seemed daunting since I had spent so many years wanting what I thought I was supposed to want.

The vastness of possibilities overwhelmed me and drove me to the comfort of my couch for a bit. Then I emerged! I began discovering that I am enough. Period. Just like that, with no buts and no fine print. All by myself, I am enough. Who knew?? Don't get me wrong, it was grueling at times: studying about self-worth and learning to manage the shame that had controlled me. I had to admit some tough stuff. Each day I uncovered more of me. I have a loving heart, I have every right to speak my voice and choose the direction of my life. I had to learn to be vulnerable! Yes, to take chances with love and life. I gained the courage to take care of ME and focus on my physical and mental health. I figured out that my job and my paycheck don't define me and I no longer need others to validate my worth.

All in all, I am quite amazed that I somehow lost myself in my work to a point that I was truly absent from my life. The beauty of this is that I have emerged with confidence, peace and the courage to be vulnerable. With these attributes I can do anything and I can do nothing. Either way I am enough! Oh, and now I can say . . . "I got fired" and I am ME because of it!

Shellie had lost herself to her career and took an honest look at the physical and emotional consequences to her and those around her. Her discovery has opened her up to fully emerge into who she is and what she wants. What more freedom can we ask for?

WEEK SIXTEEN

LIVE IN TRUTH

As we wrap up this month's theme on emergence and freedom I want to bring up a topic that is vital for a healthy world. It is the sense of inner freedom when you are true to yourself.

The Russian mystic George I. Guridieff pointed out that much of the misery that humans experience happens because we live mechanically, never properly attending to what it is to be alive. In our lives many of us hold back from being who we really are, as exemplified in Shellie's story. Have you ever noticed how many people spend years in careers that they dislike? We live our lives fearing reaction from society or consequences from our families. When we stay on the path that does not fulfill us we disconnect from part of who we are.

I understand and agree that we need to feel financially secure, but when we squelch our true talents and desires, the tradeoff of inner fulfillment is not worth the big house and expensive sports car. Please do not misunderstand; I am all for inner truth and freedom, plus a sports car and nice house—hmmm, this feels like I am on *The Price is Right*.

I enjoyed reading a book that is pertinent to this topic: *My Name is Asher Lev* by Chiam Potok. It is a story about a very religious young man who had an extraordinary talent to draw and paint. The passion that shaped his work produced fears that he would shame his religion and family. His path was difficult but he chose to pursue it. Had he not, he would have suffered the pain and anguish of living a lie.

Many of us have the belief that we should not hurt those around us. I am not advocating being self-centered by any means. What I am inviting you to think about is how fearing judgment or exclusion influences your life. People have prejudices and most of them are based on fear. This month we looked at emerging out of old behaviors and beliefs. When we resist change, we create pain for everyone involved. Every tradition wants us to behave with kindness and love but we only take this so far, as we exclude specific groups from this practice. In Week Six we talked about lovingkindness; yet when we pick and choose who we feel is deserving, we hurt ourselves and those involved.

Here is a personal story. Both my daughters are quite accomplished, brilliant, and have wonderful personalities. In her last year of college my older daughter called me and said: "Mom, we need to talk—are you sitting down?" (This was not music to my ears.) She told me she was a Lesbian. (Good that I had sat down!) I was stunned by this news and we spoke for quite some time. She asked me if I was disappointed. I thought about this question and answered, "When your sister became ill, I was disappointed in what I thought life would be like. I am not disappointed that you are gay, but I'm disappointed in the dream I had in my mind of the traditional family" (marry a nice Jewish doctor and have grandchildren), so I needed to realign my aspirations. After reading this, my daughter pointed out that this comment was not quite accurate, and I agree, so I am amending it.

Here is my addition: "We must instill in our children that gender does not matter, and they are capable of succeeding in whatever path they choose." She also reminded me that she is currently getting her doctorate, so *she* is the nice Jewish doctor! I am proud that she had and continues to have the courage to be true to herself. I never want her to feel the anguish of hiding and stifling any part of her to conform to what is deemed socially acceptable. I also told her that sexuality is only part of who she is and not to forget the she is so much more. She has a wonderful partner and I am grateful to see her embracing life fully.

It is imperative that we allow ourselves to emerge and live in truth. A funny aside—after I hung up the phone my husband asked me what we were talking about so long. We took a walk and I said: "I need to tell you something about

Jennifer." He responded: "She's pregnant." (I love the male mind.) I replied: "No, not so much…" I am grateful to be married to a man who will go where the tide leads him, and to have children who make our lives more interesting, exciting, and fulfilling.

There is a teaching in the yoga tradition I thought appropriate to share. We all have an upwelling that comes from deep within. When we discover who we really are and what we really want, there is no turning back. It is like trying to put a cap on a volcano. It creates intense pain physically, emotionally, and spiritually.

There is no escaping the reality of the cost of a rigid and closed mind. Just look at the news and you will see the impact of prejudice. Young and old are bullied for who they are or what they believe and the tension in our world is palpable. It is our reactions to what we find unacceptable that is at the root of our stress, tension, and pain—not the actual event. This is a key concept that will set you free.

Let me take this one step further. I have already spoken about the ensuing struggle in turning away from your true calling or individuality. We cause tension and hurt when we try to control others, who must live as they need to. We become stagnant when we hamper the growth and change that naturally emerge out of the twists and turns in life.

I think excerpts from the poetry book *Go In and In and In*, by Danna Faulds illustrate these concepts:

> *A life of truth walks the edge*
> *between ease and effort.*
> *There's nothing you must do*
> *to win approval, no list of*
> *saintly acts to tick off one by one,*
> *no required deprivations. Say yes*
> *to life and you are blessed with*
> *countless opportunities to choose*
> *wholeness over fragmentation. . . .*
> *Release your*

*grip on limitation, and
possibilities roll out like
endless ocean waves....*

As we close this week, I am certain that most of you are open to and accepting of others' race, gender, size, lifestyles, and sexuality. I invite you to go deeper and begin not only to tolerate difference, but to value it. It makes the world a much healthier, interesting, colorful, and spontaneous place.

In honor of this spring holiday season, while you are picking flowers or enjoying the hunt for Easter eggs, maybe along the way you can collect and embrace a few parts of yourself that you might be hiding.

Celebrate your gifts and emerge into a life of endless possibilities.

MAY

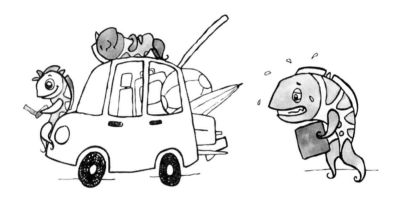

Travel

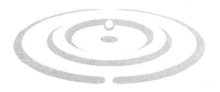

CUSTOM CALM

WEEK SEVENTEEN

VACATION TIME

It is finally here—the long-awaited vacation. You've finish packing and everyone is eager and ready to go. The road trip has begun and within a short time you cringe as you hear those dreaded words: "Are we there yet?" or "I have to go to the bathroom!" You are now officially frazzled and you are an hour into your vacation. When packing, you go to great lengths to prepare for your trip. If you are taking children, you bring out the full artillery: books, eBooks, Game Boys, iPads, movies, games, and any other electronic device to hold their attention.

Whatever happened to conversation, games with scenery, A-Z with license plates, geography, punch buggy (for those who do not know this one, you will have to know what a VW Beetle looks like), Bunny (when passing a grave yard, holding your breath—hmmm, not the best game on my list), and more. All of these have one thing in common: You have to look up, see the outside and converse with someone. Think about it—you went to great lengths to plan your family vacation, so why not enjoy time together?

The vision of our family vacation is not complete without mention of bathroom breaks. Some families try to make the trip with as few rest stops as possible. After all, isn't it worth the discomfort of a full bladder to arrive at your destination a half hour earlier? When you think about it, why the rush? It is a vacation.

Let's take a look at why we take vacations and how we show up for them. I decided to look up the true meaning of vacation and found some insight. A vacation is some period of time that we devote to pleasure and relaxation. It was also pointed out that sometimes it includes pay granted to an employee. I will focus on the first part, as pay granted to an employee might be a touchy subject.

Now, we know that our vacation is supposed to be pleasurable, restful, and relaxing. What gets in our way of embracing this time off? The main problem is that we take ourselves with us! The way we show up to life will be reflected in the way we enjoy our leisure.

We live in a world of doing and achieving, with no "off" switch. We are like the Eveready® Energizer Bunny: we keep going and going. We love our families and sincerely want to spend some quality time together, but our inability to slow down generates a level of stress.

While on vacation many of us bring along work. I remember one vacation I took when I was still in corporate America. I was working on my laptop, rather than looking at the snowcapped mountains. (Well, I was facing the window, so maybe that counts!) As I think back, I could not give myself permission to stop. After all, I thought I was needed by my job, but the reality is that none of us are that important. Many of us make the choice to sacrifice personal and family time to do work. Our behavior is that of a workaholic and even if we don't totally neglect those around us, we are still unable to just *relax.* That is a foreign word for many of us.

Yes, it is difficult to give ourselves permission for relaxation and play. Our sense of responsibility follows us everywhere we go: from planning our time off through the time we are away and then when we return.

A cover story in the *Atlanta Journal Constitution* was titled: "Just Too Ill to Chill." The article targeted pre-vacation stress and post-vacation sickness. Our immune system is impacted by stress and it can lead to getting us run down and sick, causing us to miss our vacation or get sick after we get back. The research shows that it is not the vacation that gets us sick, but the stress we incur leading up to it.

How do we escape this? (Hmmm, total retirement sounds like a good idea.) First of all, we need a shift in perspective. The vacation does not have to begin when we leave the driveway. We can take pleasure in the entire process.

- **Planning the trip:** Include whoever is participating, so everyone has a voice. Let your office know the definition of vacation. (You can cut and paste from this article.) Give yourself re-entry time when you return.
- **Packing for the trip:** Pack for yourself and help the children. No packing for spouses. I used to do this until I packed two left sneakers for my size 7 EEEE husband. (No, it was not intentional.) Of course he could not find that size in a store and from then on he packed for himself.
- **Traveling to your destination:** If you are without children, you and your partner can listen to a book you both enjoy, and then talk about it. If you are with children, of course, you want them occupied but engage with them as well. Make sure you take your time and allow for plenty of pit stops; it makes for a much more enjoyable trip.
- **While on vacation:** If you are on a getaway without the children, do not keep calling them. They will survive your absence and probably are having their own vacation. If you have to check work messages, do it when you are by yourself, (not while ordering at a restaurant) and only do this once a day. If you choose to bring work, plan to work during down time. The rest of the day, stay present with those you are with and fully engage with what you are doing. Give yourself permission to relax and play.
- **Returning home:** The trip home is still part of the vacation, so treat it that way. It's possible to be worn out from travel. When you open your door, take a breath and as you move back into your daily life, take some "vacation time." Actually, you should take some vacation time *each* day. That way you won't be waiting months in advance for the long- awaited time off.

These simple tips will make a marked difference in your entire vacation experience. Don't forget to enjoy the entire process and have fun.

Bon voyage!

WEEK EIGHTEEN

IMPACT OF TRAVEL: THE BODY

One aspect of travel that warrants special attention is the physical impact of sitting for long periods of time.

When we sit in the car, plane, office, or anywhere else, our low back can become compromised. Many techniques help relieve physical pain, but we need something we can do on the spot to target these two areas: the sacrum and hip crease. We learned earlier that the sacrum is the flat bone at the base of your spine above your tailbone and below your waist, but we need a little explanation about the hip crease. The hip crease is that spot between the abdomen and the legs, that when you sit down is "creased" near your hip joint. As I write this, the ache in my hip crease is reminding me that I have been sitting too long, so I am off for a quick break to stretch.

It is challenging to be at our best when we are uncomfortable, so here is some useful information to help you understand what tightens you up and loosens you up:

For the sacrum: It is effective to sit with your sacrum lengthened upward because it helps elongate your spine. When your sacrum is rounded back it produces tension in your low back and between your shoulder blades. You need lower-back support, but many seats do not have appropriate lumber support, which is problematic on long trips. Making your seat more comfortable can go a long way towards helping avoid unnecessary strain.

Airlines used to offer blankets, which made great low back props. I recommend bringing a small towel or soft garden pad on the plane to ensure you have something to use. Fold the blanket and place the bottom edge so it is touching your seat (you can even tuck it a bit under your bottom) and the rest goes behind your sacrum, lengthening it upward. You do not want too much lift, but just enough to make sure you do not round your back.

For the short hip crease: Many of us spend a lot of time sitting at home or the office and when we stand up we are achy. The seated position creates a forward bend at the hip crease which shortens it, generating tension in the low back. When we try to stand we find it difficult to straighten up.

Try this simple technique to help stretch out your hip crease. This is also effective for those who have limited mobility and use a walker.

- Stand up and on either side hold onto something, with your hands placed under your shoulders.
- Stand with your feet facing forward hip-width apart or narrower.
- Step your left foot forward and your right foot backward the same distance. If this hurts your lower back, take a smaller step.
- Draw your navel in toward your spine, as if you were trying to zip tight jeans. (Not that any of us has ever had to suck in our belly to do this!)
- While continuing to hold onto either side slowly bend at the hip and knee to bring your left knee over your left ankle (no further), keeping your right heel pressed into the floor.
- Stand erect. It is important to keep your shoulders over your ribs and your ribs over your hips, not forward of your hips. Keep your hips square.
- You will feel a stretch in your back hip crease and maybe into your calf. Remember to pay attention to your body and do not overdo it.
- Take a few breaths and come back to center; notice the difference and do the other side.

Waiting

I would be remiss if I did not include this next aspect of travel: waiting! We travel and do not move; we wait and wait and wait. We wait in line, on hold, in traffic—and it feels like a big waste of time. As we wait, we react to the traffic, the company that has us on hold, the clerk at the market, all causing us unnecessary anxiety. Our blood pressure and heart rate increase, our neck and shoulders tighten, our breathing gets shallow.

How can we stop this cycle? Let's take a look at two areas, body and mind.

To take care of your body: When we stand around we usually do not notice how much we tighten and strain our body. This is the opportunity to become aware and lean through your bones. Our skeleton is designed for support and when we are properly aligned we bear weight into our bones, allowing our muscles to relax. It is the same concept as lifting weights —it helps strengthen our bones.

To quiet your mind: When we react to waiting, we bring tension into both body and mind. Learning to get still and be at ease with waiting brings us into the moment and gives us the opportunity to fill up and reconnect with ourselves.

My friend had this recent experience. She was in line behind a mother and her grown children who were purchasing a cartful of clothing while chatting with the cashier. She felt her frustration grow and decided to take an easy breath. She centered herself and took it a step further. She had an extra coupon and handed it to these strangers, saving them $130.00. They were excited and grateful, and offered to take her to lunch! Because she calmed down, she was able to do something kind for someone, uplifting everyone involved.

This following simple technique will help calm your mind while taking the strain off your body:

- Stand with your feet parallel to one another, no more than hip-width apart with your spine upright. If you can spread your toes, do so. If seated, bring your feet under your knees.
- Bring your awareness to the connection to your feet on the floor and notice the distribution of your weight.
- Look straight ahead with a soft gaze.
- Check in: Is there more weight in front of your feet, or in your heels? Is the weight even? See if you can bring a bit more weight onto the front of your feet, while feeling the connection of your feet on the floor. You might notice that one side connects differently from the other.
- Now notice if your ribs are over your hips and keep your ribcage lifted.
- Notice if your head is forward. If it is, see if you can bring it back a bit.
- Now, imagine a plumb line dropping from above, through the center of your skull, continuing through the inside of your spine, through your pelvic floor, between your legs and landing between the arches of your feet.
- Take an easy inhale, then exhale as you focus your awareness on maintaining the balance in your body, feeling your feet evenly on the earth as you continue with easy breathing.

This week, practice these techniques while traveling and notice if it helps with discomfort and frustration. You will be surprised at how these few simple tools will make travel and wait time much easier on your body. If you find that you still get annoyed while you wait, don't give up. Any change takes time. Rest assured, you will have a lifetime to practice!

WEEK NINETEEN

IMPACT OF TRAVEL: THE MIND

No matter where we travel, transportation of some kind is required. We depend upon this convenience to take us where we need to go, affording us autonomy (thank goodness for GPS). Why am I focusing on this subject? The reality is that our transportation goes beyond taking us from place to place. It supplies us many opportunities to practice calming our reaction to stress and frustration. We can learn the art of patience; sometimes quickly, sometimes slowly, sometimes never!

Week Eighteen looked at the stress on our body and now our focus will be on our mind. The two are difficult to separate. Philip Chesterfield says "I find, by experience, that the mind and the body are more than married, for they are most intimately united; and when one suffers, the other sympathizes . . . " Keep in mind that although my focus is on mental tension, your body is with you so it, too, will be impacted.

Let's look at a few areas where travel can influence our mindset. Air travel is a great place to begin.

Hurry Up and Wait
My neighbor relayed this story:

> I rushed to the airport so I would have ample time before my flight. After getting through the check-in line with time to spare (a small miracle), I slowly walked to my gate. The flight boarded a little late and here I calmly sit on the plane, now an hour and a half behind schedule for takeoff. New announcement: Flight delayed another two hours so please deplane. To catch another flight I hurried off the plane to make another

flight and when I returned home I realized I had left my power cord. (I suggested that he thank the airline for giving him the opportunity to brush up on his patience and the ability to let go of attachment!)

Travel Overload

I was at the airport boarding my plane. There was a frustrated mom in front of me who was raising her voice at her child standing next to her, while holding her heavy carry-on in one hand and her baby in the other. My knee jerk reaction was disapproval of how she was speaking to her child. After all, her child was probably tired and overwhelmed.

I took a breath and chose to practice compassion, our February focus. I thought back to when my children were young, realizing I raised my voice to my children when I was frustrated. I asked her if she needed help—she did not hesitate to say *"Yes."* Her voice was still curt but she said a quick thanks. I decided to let go of my attachment to her response (I thought a big smile and hearty thank you would have been nice) and treat her with compassion, as a human being no different from myself.

We travel this world together and there are many opportunities to practice kindness. Judgment and frustration produce tension and agitation, which nobody needs. Showing kindness fosters a calm and centered state of being.

This week would not be complete without talking about driving. Air travel is basic training for travel by car. Traffic, aggressive drivers, "slow as molasses" drivers, school buses, funeral processions, and road construction are facts of life in the world of driving. We are lucky if we do not get them all on the same trip! It's upsetting, especially when we're in a hurry. Before we realize it our breathing is shallow and we feel our neck and shoulders tense up. We secretly wish we had a beat up old car so we can gently (or not so gently) nudge the car in front of us who just cut us off. This reminds me of the following common frustration we all share:

I was leaving a parking lot, planning to make a right hand turn. Much to my dismay, a car pulled out of a lot across the street and rudely blocked my entire lane, causing a lineup of cars behind me. My immediate reaction was irritation and frustration at how inconsiderate the driver was. Please understand that I expect that any of us could be frustrated by inappropriate behavior. The key is to notice it is happening so you can make a choice to do something to shift back to the here and now.

Try these two practices.

1. **Kindness:** Yes, it can be done on the road. Allow someone to merge in front of you. Seems simple, but when you are not in a good mood it is challenging. It will help change your emotional state.
2. **Breathing Technique:** This can be used on-the-spot to calm down and center yourself.
    - Take a moment to see if you are holding your breath. (I guarantee you will be if you're angry.)
    - Notice if you are tensing your neck and shoulders.
    - Now, feel the connection of your feet and, if you are driving, notice your contact to the seat beneath you.
    - Next, you are going to sigh. Start by inhaling and exhaling the first breath with an audible sound (you know it if you have teenagers) while allowing your body to soften. After the sigh, momentarily stay with the pause at the end.
    - You are not holding your breath; you are simply noticing the space at the end of the sigh. Think of a swing. After it goes up, there is a moment of stillness before it comes back down. That is your breath, and you are observing it.

- Do this a total of three times (only once if you are moving in traffic), each time staying with the pause a few moments longer, without straining. Check in on your emotional state and notice if your body is more relaxed.

Travel is a fact of life. You can use it as an opportunity to practice both kindness and this simple breath. If you practice this with the small inconveniences in life, you will have the skill to calm from the inside-out when the real challenges present themselves, It takes some getting used to, but it is worth the ride!

WEEK TWENTY

ENJOY THE JOURNEY

The most important trip of all is the journey inward.

Stephen Levine is a poet, author, and teacher. He said: "Buddha left a road map, Jesus left a road map, Krishna left a road map, Rand McNally left a road map. But you still have to travel the road yourself..."

He makes a good point. Let's look at this a little closer, beginning with our spiritual leaders. A *New York Times* article featured the originator and master teacher of a popular yoga school. He was loved, admired, and trusted by many until he behaved inappropriately with some of his female students. His sexual indiscretions caused many to leave the tradition. He is not the first spiritual leader to fall from grace.

We tend to put our spiritual leaders on pedestals, expecting them to live up to what they teach. This is not unreasonable, but we forget they are human and even if they are spiritually evolved they still can fail us with sometimes shocking behavior.

Disappointment and hurt result when we become dependent on another, expecting them to give us all of the answers. When a teacher imparts practices and teaches us to look within, then they are truly teaching and empowering. One of my most beloved teachers recently passed away and I am eternally grateful for her example of living her teachings. She taught me to go inward for my direction and strength. I tell my students: "Get dependent on the teachings, not the teacher. The practices will not fail you, but as a human being, the teacher can."

It's important to gain more clarity about the teachings, so we are able to integrate them into our daily lives. Let's take a look at a topic we can all relate to: food.

So much of our lives revolve around food. We eat so we can sustain our physical bodies, but I do not for a minute believe anyone reading this book eats for that reason alone. Food offers us a variety of choices, each containing unique tastes, textures, and smells—we eat for pleasure.

Picture this: It is late afternoon and you ate an early lunch. Hunger pains remind you that a healthy snack would be nice, so you set out to buy a piece of fruit to tide you over until dinner. As you walk through town there is a tantalizing aroma coming from the bakery across the street. Your feet go in that direction even though you are determined to walk straight home. Your mind steps in: "Should I or shouldn't I?" Too late—you are already in the bakery and your mouth is watering. The selection is wonderful and you pick out a piece of apple strudel, telling yourself that it is okay because you are still eating fruit. You are determined to take only a few bites and save the rest for dessert later on. Oops . . . you just devoured the last morsel and your hunger is satisfied . . . for the moment.

Does this sound at all familiar?

One yoga teaching says it best: "Knowledge is food; pure knowledge is the only real nourishment, that which gives satisfaction."

The strudel only satisfied your hunger for a short while. The question is, "What are we really hungry for?" We are not quite certain, so in our quest to satisfy our longing, our minds grasp onto whatever it can. It chews on the same old stuff: fears, frustrations, relationships—any person, place, or thing. There might even be a measure of satisfaction in some of these things. But it doesn't stop—it replays the same tapes over and over again.

You want answers. In your quest for more, you might take a class, study, buy a book, and speak with others, anything to attain knowledge. But no matter how hard you try, you are never satisfied. It is like an itch that must be scratched. What is this itch? It is a yearning to know more and it isn't about intellect—it cannot be found in books.

(Okay, maybe this one.) Yes, you can read others' experiences but you cannot think your way into them. Many people try this, though! Just take a look at the self-help section in any bookstore. It is massive. What is everyone looking for? Maybe this person, or that one, can help me feel better; row after row of books seem to have the answer. Or do they?

Those answers are deep within. It is in the inner stillness where you feel that sweet connection, and it is quite profound. We all have had those moments, but how do we journey inward on our own?

Meditation holds the key. When you meditate you will begin to experience something deeper than your thoughts alone. You will move from the externalities to your own inner depth and strength. It's like the pastry from the bakery.

You can describe the aroma, flavor, and feeling that you get as you took the first bite, but you cannot truly convey your experience—that must be done on our own. Once you know, you know, and you will begin to live from this place of deeper understanding. When you forget, you only need to quiet your mind to remember. The parts of you that keep you stuck will melt away and your hunger will be fed from within.

There are many meditation techniques, and some are scattered throughout this book. It is helpful to begin with a breathing practice as a gateway into meditation. I like Alternate Nostril Breathing because it gives your mind a specific focus to jump-start you into meditation. Additionally, it helps to revitalize the nervous system and balance the brain hemispheres.

- Use your thumb for one side and the ring and pinky fingers for the other side. You can tuck the other two fingers. Keep the inhalation even with the exhalation.
- Close off the right nostril with your thumb and slowly inhale through the left nostril for the count of four.

- Close off the left nostril with your ring and pinky fingers and slowly exhale through the right nostril for the count of four. Then slowly inhale through the right nostril for the count of four.
- Close off the right nostril with your thumb and slowly exhale through the left nostril for the count of four. Then slowly inhale through the left nostril for the count of four.
- Continue this sequence for a total of five rounds and end with the exhalation through your left nostril.
- Sit for a few minutes and if your thoughts surface, focus on your breathing.

The point is to use the breath as a vehicle to take you to the stillness within. If you get momentary glimpses of quiet, you have gotten a lot from the practice. Work your way up to practicing daily for five minutes. (Of course, you can go longer.) When you try to quiet your mind, you realize just how busy it is. It loves to be entertained!

Please be tolerant and gentle with the process. It only takes a few minutes of daily practice to begin the most exquisite journey of all: traveling inward to the space of peace. You have everything you need for this trip and there is no passport required.

Enjoy the journey.

JUNE

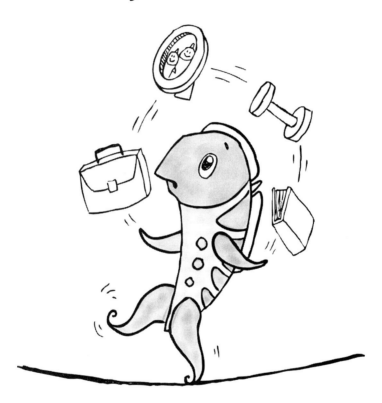

Balanced Living

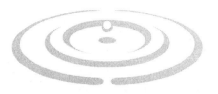

CUSTOM CALM

WEEK TWENTY-ONE

ACTIVITY

An important aspect of balanced living is exercise and movement. There is no need to feel guilty if you are not one who goes to the gym and works up a sweat. I, for one, have resisted the urging of my family to participate in this way, as heavy sweating is not for me. The intention of exercise is to keep your body and mind healthy and fit. Since we all have different abilities, limitations, and needs, we need to stay open to possibilities other than very active workouts. (Buns of steel and six-pack abs are not part of this equation.) Let's begin with a few articles that support exercise of all kinds.

The Wall Street Journal's January 5, 2010, article titled "The Hidden Benefits of Exercise" emphasizes how all activity, including moderate exercise, produces positive effects on both the immune system and chronic diseases.

The New York Times' August 1, 2011, article titled "Ancient Moves for Orthopedic Problems" focuses on the benefit of many yoga practices for those with joint problems or osteoporosis. The beauty of some yoga practices is that they do not stress the joints, yet they strengthen the bones.

We know that there is much research and data supporting exercise, and I bring this up with the intention of opening the door for many possibilities.

I am in no way negating the benefits of sweating and cardio, but many people need other options. When I began to exercise, I had Lupus, so high-impact exercise was not appropriate. I needed to find other avenues that were effective for my body and mind.

One of my clients has developed arthritis in her spine so she is no longer able to exercise as she once did. The deep yoga practice she enjoyed has been replaced with other forms of exercise. Gardening is one of her activities that helps sustain both her body and mind. Over time, as our bodies change, so do our needs. What might have been beneficial over the years may need to shift to accommodate the different conditions of the body.

When I have visited traditional gyms, I notice most people rush out right after exercising with little or no stretching. Many do not understand that this is not healthy for your muscles. Whether you work out, play golf, play tennis, garden, or engage in any other activity, your muscles contract and tighten which decreases their blood supply. Taking the time to do some simple stretches has tremendous value. It will lengthen your muscles, allowing more blood and oxygen to keep them healthy.

When you stretch out keep this in mind:

- Treat stretching back out as part of your workout and budget the extra time into your practice.
- Direct your breath into the area that is tight.
- Have something to support you while stretching; for example, lean against a bench or wall.
- Do not overstretch where you feel pain; you cannot relax into pain and you will intensify the tension.
- Stay with the stretch for a few breaths and allow the muscles you are lengthening to slowly release.

The following quote by Chungliang Al Huang is a great introduction to the next aspect of healthy living: "Many people treat their bodies as if they were rented from Hertz—something they are using to get around in but nothing they genuinely care about understanding . . ." I am not advocating that we need to all go back to school and learn anatomy. What I notice is that many of us are not aware of our bodies until we are in pain. Please understand that your body needs your attention so you can make choices about how to effectively use and maintain it.

Let's begin with why abdominals are so important. (Yes, they are in there somewhere). I see many people doing all sorts of abdominal workouts but do not know how to use their abs efficiently when they are out and about. Abdominals support and stabilize your spine and specific abdominal muscles help decrease tension in your lower spine while others lengthen your upper spine.

The *transverse* abdominal muscles help you lengthen your lower spine. They are the weaker abdominal muscles and can be difficult to isolate. If you drilled a hole through your body an inch below your navel (this is not to be taken literally), you will land at the top of your sacrum. When you draw the transverses in, they will help lengthen your sacrum, reducing low back compression. We touched on this in the week on back pain.

To begin to isolate the transversus muscles and learn to use your legs at the same time, try this every time you get up or sit down on a chair:

- Scoot forward on your seat with your feet a little behind your knees.
- Slowly draw your navel in and up to use your abdominal muscles.
- Hinge at your hip joint, leaning your upper body forward, keeping your abdominals engaged.
- Press through your legs, keeping a bit more weight in the front of your feet, and get up slowly without pulling up with your back muscles. You can place your hands on your thighs for support. Lead more from your chest. Focus on isolating your abdominals to support your spine while using your legs.
- Now, from standing, keep your abdominals engaged, press into your legs, hinge at the hips and lead yourself down with your sitting bones (butt first), and slowly sit down. (No plunking!)

*For those with knee problems, be mindful that you are not straining your knees.

As you practice, you will discover how to effectively isolate your abdominals and legs for support rather than straining your body with every movement. Think about how many times a day you get up and down from a chair, or walk up steps. You can be giving your abs and legs a workout simply by using them efficiently.

Remember to take care of your body and give it the exercise and attention it deserves. You will be the beneficiary of increased strength and stamina when you choose a practice that meets your specific physical and emotional needs. After all, this is the only body you have, and since there are no returns or trade-ins, keep it tuned up!

WEEK TWENTY-TWO

LIVING LIFE FULLY

Week Twenty-One shed some light on the importance of taking care of your body to live a more balanced life. Let's shift the focus to a different kind of balanced living, one of living life with greater awareness and clarity.

In the play *Hamlet*, his question was: "To be or not to be?" That is the question I will ask here. Are we human beings, or human doings? Okay, I am full of short queries, but they really do invite you to explore how you show up for life.

Let me begin with the experience of taking our pointer for a walk. (Actually, she walks us.) My husband takes her in the early morning (kudos to him—I am in my warm bed) and I take her in the late afternoon. She would much rather take walks than run around in the yard, and now I understand why. She is absolutely amazed by bunny rabbits. We are both awestruck by her ability to completely focus on what she sees, especially bunnies. (Sad but true—since the kids are grown, this is what we talk about.)

There are a few houses on our route that consistently have bunnies in their yards. When she spots one, she stops, lifts her front paw, and straightens her tail. No matter what else is happening around her she stays in full point, just staring until we notice. Then she will move forward slowly, without disturbing the bunny. She takes one little step at a time, stopping in between.

Sometimes, I want her to walk more quickly toward the rabbit, but she is unmovable. She teaches me about complete focus. The ability to be absorbed in the moment is a lifelong practice. For the pointer, it is a natural instinct, but for humans I think we need to constantly remind ourselves to notice what is around us.

Now, when we pass the house with the bunnies, I too focus and see if they are out. I really pay attention and am aware of details that I never saw before. I guess you can "teach an old human new tricks!"

This simple lesson reminds me of a couple of quotes. The first one is from the Robert Fulghum book written back in the mid-80s: *All I Really Need to Know I Learned in Kindergarten.* This quote is quite simple: "Be aware of wonder. Live a balanced life—learn some and think some and draw and paint and sing and dance and play and work every day some."

In the second one, Albert Einstein says: "He who can no longer pause to wonder and stand rapt in awe, is as good as dead; his eyes are closed."

In both quotes, the word *wonder* makes me think about how we live much of our lives mechanically and unaware. In April, I spoke about taking time each day to lighten up, but consider this thought: Only when we really are present can we see the simple pleasures unfolding before us.

Children today have their lives jam-packed. They go from school to other activities, staying busy from morning until night. It is a world of entertainment and rushing around, cell phones, games, and TV; we have lost the ability to be still. After a while, we no longer know who we are.

I find there is some concern about getting quiet. It seems that many equate calming down with feeling tired or being boring. I admit sometimes when you finally allow yourself to stop, you realize just how exhausted you are. Calm does not mean slow and sluggish. What I am targeting here is that when you live a calm, centered life you can feel energized at the same time. One does not preclude the other. Many of us live life on pure adrenaline—stressing, reacting, and charging forward while missing out on what we are doing. Even if you need to rush to get somewhere, you can be aware of the fact that you are rushing and feel calm at the same time. I talked about this before: allow yourself to be where your feet are planted.

Let's go back to the question—*to be or not to be?* To *be* means to exist or live, not to survive and *do*. When we are able to simply be, we live with openness, awe, and wonder. Think about babies. The first time they look at something new, they explore it using all of their senses. We could take a lesson from them.

The University of Massachusetts Medical School is the home of The Stress Reduction Clinic. The clinic's focus is on Mindful-Based Stress Reduction to help those suffering with chronic pain and stress. I participated in a training to learn the techniques employed there. One exercise required that we lie down with our backs on the floor. We were guided into Happy Baby pose, a yoga pose that helps us understand what yoga is really about. In this pose, you lie on your back and bring your legs up in the air and look and play with your toes. (That is, if you can still reach them!) We were asked to do this with curiosity and playfulness as a baby would. In case you are concerned, no, we did not have to put them in our mouth!

To begin cultivating the ability to feel calm and take in what is around you at the moment, give mindful walking a try. Keep an open mind and let go of judgment. You can do this outside and even take your shoes off.

- Walk in slow motion and notice the mechanics of walking. Place your heel on the floor, roll your foot while shifting your weight and pushing off with your back leg.
- While slowly walking, take in exactly what is in front of you. This is not sightseeing, but simply looking at what is in your line of sight. Do this for fifteen steps and then slowly turn around while looking ahead and taking in the entire panorama; then walk the other way.
- Use your senses: what do you hear, smell, see, and feel? It could be the warmth of the sun on your body, the sensation of a breeze, the fragrance of flowers, or maybe it is the shapes you see when you look at a tree.

- If you are thinking about something, notice your thoughts while still engaging your other senses. All of these things are happening at the same time.
- Now, try this at your normal cadence or even when you are rushing and see if you can maintain your focus. The key is to stay in awareness the entire time.

This practice will teach you to immerse yourself in what you are doing in the moment and see the beauty and freshness right in front of you.

No need to wait for time off to enjoy yourself. You can live a balanced life simply by paying attention. Ordinary miracles are happening around you every day—all you need to do is open your eyes and notice.

WEEK TWENTY-THREE

SLEEP

Our body needs sleep, yet so many of us complain that we are sleep deprived. Remember the sweet bedtime saying: "Good night, sleep tight and don't let the bed bugs bite?" Back then, we tightened up because we were on constant alert for the dreaded bed bugs, and this was our good night sendoff! (If you have carried on this tradition, you might want to change it up a bit.) What is wrong with this picture?

We still fight off bedbugs, but they have morphed into the constant chatter in our mind, hindering our ability to get a good night's sleep or to wake up refreshed. We drag ourselves out of bed and before we are able to be civil to those around us, we need our caffeine jolt. Whether at the convenience store or supermarket, you can find a plethora of caffeine-infested drinks with extra energy shots to get you through the day. Then, at the end of the day, we need to calm down (no wonder), so we grab a beer or glass of wine. Some take medication to get relief. It's true, we all need some perking up or calming down from time to time, but it seems many are stuck in a vicious cycle.

Sleep deprivation wreaks havoc on your body and mind. Even if you are able to fall asleep, at some point you awaken during the night. This is natural, but the problem is our inability to fall back to sleep. When I teach a program on Enhancing Sleep and Stamina, it is well attended, which underscores the need for some practical options. I hear two common struggles.

1. There is pain somewhere in the body so the mind is off and running, judging the pain and magnifying the sensation.

2. The mind will just not stop. We think ourselves into exhaustion, and even that does not help us sleep.

We ruminate over work, the kids, friends, our spouse, our parents, the shopping list, not getting enough sleep, and anything or everything that is going on in our lives. We attempt to stop our thoughts, which is like trying to stop a freight train. We need a way to engage the brakes to slowly come to a halt.

There are simple tools that can help us fall back to sleep, or at least allow our body to go into a deep state of relaxation. The following are two that I find quite helpful:

Gentle Twist

This simple spinal twist has some wonderful benefits:

- Calms your nervous system.
- Massages your internal organs, increasing their blood and oxygen supply.
- Lengthens and twists the spine.
- It is easy to do in bed, but if you are sleeping with someone, a gentle shove might be needed!

Try this:

- Lie on your back and bring your knees to your chest.
- Hold your knees and roll over to the right side, keeping your knees bent at a right angle, and allow them rest on the bed. Make sure your legs are no lower than the right angle to your torso.
- Slide your left hand to your waist and allow your elbow to rest back, creating a gentle twist to your spine. If your knees come apart, or if you feel too much pull, place a pillow or your hand between your knees.

- Rest your head wherever it is most comfortable.
- Stay here for 2-4 minutes noticing your breath; then change sides.

*If this hurts in any way, come out of the pose. If you have any disc problems or any form of osteoporosis, you must be extra careful as any deep twisting may be counterproductive.

Breath

I talk about breath often because it is paramount to maintaining a healthy body. When a baby breathes, its entire body moves like a little accordion. As we age, our breath gets constricted, limiting our oxygen intake.

Focused, deep breathing will promote sleep in two ways. First, it will give you a way to anchor your mind into the present moment. Second, you will begin to oxygenate your body and foster a state of deep relaxation.

Try the following exploration that breaks down breath into three parts:

Start by lying on your back. If you like, place a pillow under your knees. Then put one hand on your belly and the other on your ribcage to help you notice if the breath is getting into the specific areas.

Part 1: Belly—Lower Lobes of Your Lungs

- Without force or effort, inhale while expanding the abdomen as much as is comfortable, as if you were filling a balloon. Do this without expanding the ribcage.
- At the end of the inhalation, your navel will be at its most extended point.

- When exhaling, your abdomen moves inward. At the end of the exhalation give your belly a gentle squeeze inward.
- Continue for a few more breaths and then return to your natural breath.

Part 2: Ribcage—Middle Lobes of Your Lungs

- Discontinue using your abdomen with your breath and begin to inhale and exhale slowly as you direct your breath into your ribcage.
- Notice the expansion of your ribcage as you gently inhale. Your sides and back may expand as well.
- Exhale by relaxing your chest muscles. Notice your ribcage contracting as the air exits your lungs.
- Breathe slowly into your chest with total awareness, without using your belly.
- Continue for a few more breaths and then return to your natural breath.

Part 3: Collarbones and Clavicle—Upper Lobes of Your Lungs

- Inhale directly into your ribcage once again and expand your breath a bit more into the upper portion of your lungs around the base of your neck. Your shoulders and collar bones will probably move up slightly, which will take a bit of effort.
- Exhale slowly, first releasing your lower and upper chest, then relaxing the rest of the ribcage back to its starting position.
- Continue for a few more breaths and then return to your natural breath.

Part 4: The Entire Three-Part Breath

- Feel the air reaching into the bottom of your lungs.
- At the end of abdominal expansion, start to expand through your chest: front, back, and sides.
- When your ribs are fully expanded, inhale a bit more until you feel the expansion in the upper portion of your lungs around the base of your neck, without forcing the breath. Your body remains in a relaxed state. This completes one inhalation.
- Exhale, first through your upper breathing area, then your ribcage, and then your belly. At the end, give your belly a gentle squeeze.
- Continue this breathing, without straining in any way. Allow it to be as natural as possible.

As you practice, you will begin to notice how effective your breathing is (if you are alive, it is somewhat effective). You will find the areas of your body where breath is limited, and that is where yoga and stretching is beneficial. Please do not force the breath into tight areas because that will agitate your mind, which would defeat the purpose. Simply notice the breath and allow it to be easy. If this practice is difficult for you, become aware of your breath in a more generalized way or go back to one of the techniques mentioned earlier in the book.

Anything that helps you relax and ward off the bedbugs of your mind is worth a try. In the meantime, I bid you a bedtime farewell: "Good night, sleep loosely, and immerse into tranquility."

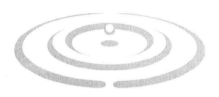

CUSTOM CALM

WEEK TWENTY-FOUR

BALANCE FROM THE INSIDE-OUT: DIANE'S STORY

There are times when life takes an unexpected turn and we are thrown off balance. Situations arise and they shape our lives in a way that we never would have imagined. We have a choice whether to learn from them and evolve, or shut down.

Many people who inspire us have overcome tremendous obstacles and developed more strength and wisdom than they had before. This quote describes it well: "We are all faced with a series of great opportunities brilliantly disguised as impossible situations." – Charles R. Swindoll. I will dive deeper into this topic later in the book, but I bring it up here because sooner or later we are all faced with difficulties that perpetuate new growth. (When this happens, I call it another @!%&*# growth opportunity!)

Diane's touching story poignantly illustrates her evolution:

> Having had breast cancer changed my life! That sounds so cliché. I know it "changes" everyone who currently has or has had any type of cancer, but for me it brought balance into my very unbalanced life. I can't explain the day I sprang from the darkness into the sunlight, but I'd say it was somewhere after the chemotherapy and before the re-growth of my hair. Let me explain.
>
> My story begins like many others. I was raised as a middle class child, went to college, and then moved to Atlanta to pursue my dream. My dream had always been to live in a big city, own a home, and be self-sufficient. But I had difficulty setting down roots in the big city and found it challenging to make friends; so af-

ter four years I returned to the comfort of my hometown. I firmly believe that our reactions to change can exacerbate diseases. The stresses of changing my lifestyle unveiled a disease that had been lying dormant since childhood.

After years of testing and countless visits to doctors, I was misdiagnosed with multiple sclerosis. I felt like I was handed a death sentence and feared I was going to have to rearrange my entire life. While growing up, I was not what anyone would call a very graceful child. Some things never change, as I am in my late forties and still am not what you would call a very graceful adult!

It was not until I returned to Atlanta, went to Emory University, and underwent additional testing, that I was properly diagnosed. I have hereditary cerebellar degeneration. The main symptom I live with every day is ataxia, which is another word for irregular gait. Having little balance makes life tricky. Learning to deal with the silent stares and the hushed snickers can be demeaning and discouraging until you realize that it comes from others' lack of knowledge of the disease. Someone once told me, "What other people think about you is none of your business." That resonated with me and struck many chords. The disease is progressive and the symptoms could get much worse. This was my new normal.

Ten years later, out of nowhere, I was diagnosed with Stage I breast cancer. From the moment I heard the doctor say the words, "unfortunately, the test came back positive . . . ," I decided I was not going to let this finding be another death sentence, as was hearing I had ataxia. I had lived through a very dark time dealing with the first diagnosis. But, by faith and encouragement from my parents and friends, I pulled myself back into the light and began looking at life optimistically again. Even though I was still living, and will always live, with ataxia, I was determined to not let the cancer diagnosis bring me down. I figured the only thing I could control was my attitude. I decided to meet each day with humor. I kept a twinkle in my eye when I felt like crying and a smile on my face when I felt nauseous from the chemo. Since I am an avid swimmer, I would kid and say my new breast implants would keep me afloat in the water. This helped me minimize the fear I felt.

After my mastectomy, chemotherapy, reconstruction, and even tattoos, I was introduced to a new normal, yet again. The change in my body's physical appearance, coupled with the fact that the chemotherapy threw me straight into menopause, was trying, to say the least. On the outside, I appeared fine and the threat of cancer was gone, but still I struggled. The ataxia, which had gotten worse from the chemo, remained my constant companion. As I have progressed through life, I have learned to take care of myself with a renewed attitude of optimism and a daily choice to live in the light.

It has been said that every adversity leads you to a better place, and it has. There is a translation in a religious text that is meaningful to me: "I was given the gift of a handicap. At first I didn't think of it as a gift, and begged God to remove it. And then He told me, 'My grace is enough, it's all you need. My strength comes into its own in your weakness.' "

I quit focusing on the handicap and started appreciating the gift... Now I take limitations in stride, and with good cheer... And so the weaker I get, the stronger I become. Every day, instead of waiting for the other shoe to drop, I just put one shoe in front of the other as I walk one day at a time, living my life with a spring in my step and my head held high. For me, that is all the balance I need to enjoy life.

No matter what disability, illness, or challenge you face, you can choose to progress toward your full capacity as a human being. Diane went through a dark time in her life, but emerged with a balanced attitude and outlook. Balance is more than making sure your work, play, exercise, and social life keep you on an even keel. Being in balance also does not mean that you will not sometimes feel saddened or frustrated by what you have on your plate. Balance is the ability to spring back into symmetry, regroup, and move forward. You will constantly have to realign yourself as you go off course; this is a fact of life. Diane's capacity to find equilibrium on the inside accurately and sensitively conveys the meaning of balance.

JULY

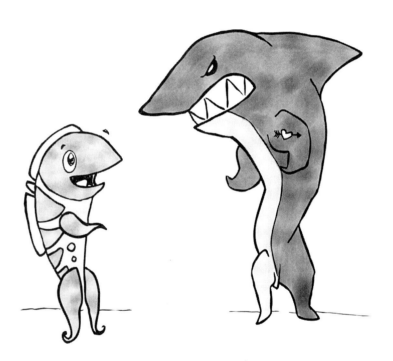

Relationships & Emotions

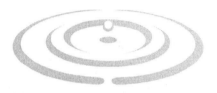

CUSTOM CALM

WEEK TWENTY-FIVE

UN-HOOK FROM REACTION

Relationships and emotions need to be explored together because they are so intertwined. In relationships, we often seem to be at the mercy of our emotions, feeling a little out of control; but we don't have to be. The following quote will help shine some light on the subject: "When you feel yourself in the grip of an emotion such as jealousy or anger or sorrow ... take a step back ... You can allow the emotion to run through you without causing negative thoughts or actions." Gary Zukov.

After reading this, you might think something like, "You have got to be kidding; there is no way to take a step back when I want to confront a situation. After all, I have the right to feel how I am feeling." You're right; it's a challenge for all of us. The two categories of action are markedly different: the Response versus the Knee-Jerk reaction.

Response
We all interact within many relationships: family, friends, strangers, and institutions. Inevitably there will be a confrontation or hurt feelings. Responding occurs from the present moment. We gain the ability to see a situation clearly because we have disengaged and observed what has happened. This takes some of the charge out of it. We can respond when we are more neutral and do not take the situation personally, even if the behavior of others is hurtful.

Knee-Jerk Reaction
The topic of knee-jerk reaction could fill volumes on its own—we all have plenty of experiences to contribute. When we react, we display a behavior or emotion following an incident. Sometimes, our reaction propels us into appropriate action, but often it generates problems. Most of the time when we get angry or hurt, it is because we take things personally. We get

into trouble when we demonstrate negatively charged knee-jerk reactions that generate anxiety and stress. We get hooked and react, which not only takes us out of the moment but compromises our physical and emotional well-being. Our reaction bubbles up because we are either in the past or future; not in the present moment.

When we consider our relationships, we know how wonderful and rich they can be, and we also are aware of their challenges. Those we care about the most can easily frustrate us—our significant other, our business associates, our children, or our parents. I once heard someone talking about how her parents really push her buttons. Another person replied, "Remember, they installed them."

How do we uninstall these buttons? (I think some of them are SuperGlued.) At the very least, how do we stop them from derailing us? Emotions are part of our nature and they are meant to be felt, but when we allow them to take over we create problems. In my work with those affected by stress, pain, and illness, I find two consequences that arise when we remain in reaction:

1. *We become our reactions.* We express how we feel as "I am angry" or "I am sad" rather than saying, "I feel angry" or "I feel sad." These are very different. If you are the emotion, then you have lost any choice and the inappropriate knee-jerk reaction will follow. The feeling needs to be felt and then you can move on.
2. *We are not able to see clearly.* Most of our reactions are based on our past experience. Only when you take a step back and view the situation without layering your judgments and perceptions will the emotion no longer have a grip on you. You can see with greater clarity the situation in its own context and bring yourself back to the here and now.

Many times the feelings are justified, but the problem arises when our behavior is inappropriate. Yelling, stomping, gossiping, and name-calling are harmful to both you and those around you, and your knee-jerk reactions can lead to these behaviors in a flash. It is like being blindsided by a car. You don't see it coming until it is too late, after the damage is done.

How can you step on the brakes instantly so you can respond appropriately? Here are some simple tools to accomplish that:

- Visualize a Stop Sign in your mind. (Not a Right-of- Way, but Stop.)
- Feel your feet connecting to the earth.
- Notice your heartbeat.
- Take a few breaths until your belly relaxes. I repeat this simple tool because it is vital, easy, and accessible.
- Walk away (not stomp) and tell the person you will talk later. If you cannot speak calmly, then simply walk away slowly.
- Bring to mind someone you care about (it may be the person you are reacting to) and remember the feelings evoked.
- Bring to mind how you feel when you are being yelled at. This is very powerful and can stop you in your tracks.

What do all of these tools have in common? They bring you back to the present moment. Any one of the above suggestions will give you the pause needed to come back to the moment and respond appropriately. They will help you live with more ease and are certain to improve your relationships. Your need to apologize will diminish, and that in itself is worth the effort. Even if you felt the other person deserved this reaction, think about what you are doing to your own body and mind. It is not worth the momentary rush of pleasure.

Bring to mind a previous altercation in which you were involved. If you are having trouble thinking of one, remember the last time you were on the phone with customer service!

Review the situation and notice a few things: Were you able to really hear what the other person was saying or were you planning your response? Did you raise your voice and talk at the person? Was your heart beating faster, your breath shorter? Whether you remember or not, each one of these symptoms stems from the fact that you had a knee-jerk reaction.

If you slip up and inappropriately react to another and later realize that you should have used one of the above quick interventions, you are already on your way to change—you are aware of your behavior. Give one of these a try and see which quick technique works best for you, or maybe you can come up with one from your personal experience. Remember, this shift will take time.

I designed these tools to be easy and practical because we need something quick and effective to avert the impending train wreck. There are many techniques and perspectives throughout this book that, over time, will help you transform your reactions into responses. Who knows? Maybe next year when you read this book, you will be able to skip this section!

WEEK TWENTY-SIX

PERSONALITY TRAITS

Many personality traits underlie our reactions toward others. We have had some of them for decades, so it is easy to be unaware of their impact. They can create anxiety and stress while undermining our relationships and wellbeing. After careful consideration, I came up with two traits that I feel are quite common. If you do not relate to these, then consider traits that are more obvious for you.

Stubbornness

Many of us are stubborn. At times, it can be a positive characteristic because it gives us perseverance when we need it. However, I bring this up in the section on Relationships & Emotions because often, stubbornness wreaks havoc on the body, mind, and relationships. We dig in our heels and stand our ground, leaving little room for other possibilities. There is certainly nothing wrong with having your philosophies and beliefs. It is when you get stuck in your way of thinking that you end up frustrated with others.

I grew up with a Dad who was passionate about many things in life. Much of the time this was a wonderful and inspiring way to live and we spent much of our lives reaping the benefits. However, at times his zeal to help us understand that he was correct was not as persuasive as he would have hoped. I remember years back my mother, sister, brother, and I were sitting around the dinner table and the discussion turned to politics. (Yes, a big mistake!) It was the election year of 1972. As the discussion became heated, with utmost conviction Dad said, "You vote for Nixon, or you don't vote!" We found this quite amusing knowing that he was not allowed in the voting booth with us, and my sister and I proceeded to vote for McGovern (No, we never told him and at 94, I hope when he reads this book, he will forgive us!) No matter how strong your convictions, others might not see things your way and in the process of trying to force others to believe as you do, your emotions can get the best of you.

This brings me to an important question: Would you rather be right or happy?

Some of you might answer this question with a resounding "I would rather be right!" because, after all, you know best. Even if you are correct it is not worth the cost to you and others around you. Ruminating over the situation only creates stress and anxiety. You might not have control over others' beliefs but you do have the choice to back off so you can enjoy life. Give it a chance. It's up to you.

Negativity and Guilt

Both negativity and guilt are common traits that have tremendous impacts on life. These traits involve much more than the "glass half-empty vs. half-full" scenario. A negative attitude spirals you into sluggishness and anxiety. You may remember I earlier mentioned being "slimed" with negativity. Well, we may not realize it but we may be the ones bringing the slime. We complain and focus on the negative and miss out on the opportunity for joy that is right in front of us. We hear complaining at work, at home, and throughout our day, and it becomes toxic for us, even if we are not the one being negative.

Negativity usually perpetuates guilt. (Jewish guilt does not hold the trophy. I hear every religion has its own special brand, so don't worry, no one is left out.) Guilt spirals us into negativity and we act out of tension, not out of choice. Our thoughts become destructive and we feel either angry or sad.

Most people with negative attitudes are not even aware that they are so negative. They complain constantly and wonder why they feel so stressed and sluggish.

As I write this, I am beginning to feel fatigue, so I will shift to something positive—The Solution! How to prevent our negative traits from wreaking havoc on everyone (including ourselves) and transform them into endearing aspects of our personality and individuality?

I first need to detour to a common definition of "insanity." (No, I am not calling anyone insane but after you hear more, you might decide that the shoe fits!) It means doing the same thing over and over again expecting different results.

If you are hammering something and continue to smack your thumb, you would either stop or change your approach, right? Or would you?

In our relationships we behave in the same way. Our approach may not get the results we were hoping for, yet we continue to employ them. It is difficult to change some of our ingrained ways of behaving, even when we are aware of the negative consequences.

What happens is that our mind gets stuck in our own perceptions of how things are or should be, leaving no room for other possibilities. It becomes a good, bad, right, or wrong judgment and we perpetuate our behavior.

When we are able to quiet our minds, we can take a step back and see with more clarity. Only then do we have the ability to be open and receptive to other options. Let me give you an analogy that might help. Picture a lake on a crystal-clear day. You can see your reflection while seeing what is at the bottom. A small gust of wind stirs up a few waves and you can still see but there is some distortion. Then a strong wind blows through and all you can see is murky water and debris from broken branches and leaves.

This is exactly how the mind works. We see through the filters of our personal history and beliefs about life, distorting what is really in front of us. If you have ever tried on glasses that are not your prescription, you get the idea. Our reactions and decisions are based on this distorted information.

It takes practice to see what is actually occurring beyond the stories in our minds. To become more aware, give this a try:

- Stand or sit down and look at what is directly in front of you. Describe what you see. It works well to either go outside or look through a window.
- Now, describe it again without using any name to identify it. Do this with no subjective adjectives; for example, do not say, "I see a pretty flower." Someone else might not see it as pretty. You can say something like, "I see petals that are a medium yellow, with a few shades of brown throughout."
- If you catch yourself shading what is there with your personal history, come back to what you really see. For example; if you are looking at a sofa and it reminds you of Aunt Lilly's sofa you will now have an opinion based on your memory of your Aunt. How can you describe it without that memory or that opinion? And how has your response changed?

This exercise will help illustrate how much of what you see is through your personal history and filters, which stem from thoughts. As you practice, you will begin to cultivate a clearer way of seeing what is really there.

You can transform habits that do not serve you well into positive aspects of who you are: quirkiness, individuality, passion, humor, caution, curiosity, and so many more. The saying, "You don't need to throw the baby out with the bathwater" holds true here; don't throw the positive parts of your personality away, just the ones that are troublesome.

By addressing the traits that once produced stress and anxiety, you will develop a clear, calm, and effective means of interacting.

WEEK TWENTY-SEVEN

COMMUNICATION

I watched a segment on the *Today* show about annoying habits of those you are in a relationship with.

Please do not take out your pen and paper and use this as an opportunity to list the terrible habits of your children, parents, co-workers, and significant others. I am sure they all have them and am certain you have a few as well. This is not meant as an insult; after all, we are creatures of habit and there will always be behaviors that we find annoying. This is what makes relationships so entertaining!

Week Twenty-Six highlighted personality traits that can be destructive to relationships and some simple techniques to help you abort negative reactions right before chaos erupts. This week's entry is more about idiosyncrasies and exasperating habits that hinder our enjoyment of others.

One of the most difficult challenges in relationships is to let others be who they are, quirks and all, without layering our objections and reactions onto their behavior. This is quite difficult but necessary to maintain healthy and uplifting relationships.

I asked my parents what they felt was the key ingredient in sustaining their 71-year marriage. Dad's answer: "Loyalty, love and integrity. Your mom shared and enjoyed my successes. We had a lot in common. I knew she was an honorable girl." Mom's answer: "Your dad was an honest man. I gave in often. He never questioned me about what I spent and he respected my judgment. I loved him and was told to marry a man with character and I married one! Don't be swayed by glitter and glamour. We are comfortable with each other." They each have kept their individual identities as well as their sense of humor throughout their marriage, but you can see they approached it differently.

As I was writing this book, my family came up with some ideas that I have incorporated. When I mentioned this topic, they were very supportive and took the opportunity to help me see a few of my endearing quirks. First was *house-yelling*. Rather than walking to the room to say what is on my mind, I begin my sentence from another room. In fairness to me and others who have this habit, part of the reason is so I do not forget what I wanted to say. Plus, at times I am unsure of where they are and they are bound to hear me if I speak loud enough. Now, I make the effort to find them and talk about things instead of yelling.

Next was one habit about which I finally gained clarity; conversing with my spouse while he is watching television. As I spoke, I would notice his eyes looking past me to the television. I found this very frustrating, so I would leave in a huff feeling insulted that he found the television more important than a conversation with me. With practice, I now am able to see that it is not about me. It is simply about the fact that my husband is interested in what he is watching. Now, I stay in the moment and kindly ask him when would be a better time to talk.

I am sure we all have our favorite examples of annoying habits, and the question is how to modify our responses so they do not stir up problems.

I will briefly revisit the first of yoga's guidelines to our behavior, *ahimsa,* or non-harmfulness. *Ahimsa* helps deter us from causing harm stemming from our reactions. The obvious behaviors are easy to spot and amend, but even the subtle looks, tones, or comments sting the person to whom we are directing them and cause damage.

Poor communication is the main culprit. If we were aware of how much harm it causes to those we care about, we would work on changing it. There are two aspects of communication common to us all—Listening and Speaking.

Listening

There are times in conversation when we are thinking about our response before the other person is finished speaking. We interrupt, which is frustrating and dismissive to the speaker and others around us. Many times we do not even realize we are doing it. The point I want to emphasize is you cannot be present in the conversation if you are interrupting or pre-planning what you are going to say.

Here are a few tips that will help you listen more attentively:

- If it is not a good time for you to listen, kindly suggest a better time.
- While the person is speaking, feel your feet on the floor.
- Make eye contact while you are listening.
- If you feel the urge to speak, become aware of your breath as you inhale and exhale to guide yourself back to listening.
- Have a 5-second rule before you speak. (That is my husband's suggestion for me and you will be amazed at how long 5 seconds take.)
- If you are unsure about what has been said, stop and ask the person to repeat their statement. This way you will not drift into trying to figure out what you just heard.

When you attempt to tune into what another is saying you will be surprised at how challenging it is to pay full attention. To improve your listening skills you will need to cultivate your ability to rein your mind back to the present moment. All of the above suggestions will quickly and easily help you accomplish this.

Speaking

The second guideline in this yoga teaching is *satya*, or truthfulness. *Satya* invites us to speak the truth at all times. However, we must be discerning because sometimes speaking our truth can bring harm to another. How do we practice both *ahimsa* and *satya* simultaneously?

Part of the problem arises when we give advice or speak without thinking it through. This creates hurt feelings and relationship discord. There are many techniques to help with this; the following practice is simple and extremely effective.

Before speaking ask yourself these three questions:
1. Is it true?
2. Is it kind?
3. Is it necessary?

Often the first is on target, but the second and third can get a bit murky. Many of our comments are well-meaning, but unnecessary. Think about how many times you have received unsolicited advice or opinions and how it felt. Even the most innocent comment can be hurtful and uncalled for.

We have the tendency to respond to others very quickly. Taking a moment to pause and get centered before you speak will give you time to ask yourself if what you were about to say is appropriate. Listening attentively and mindfully will cultivate your ability to do this.

This week, give these suggestions a try. Did you hold back on a comment? Did you notice when you made an unnecessary comment? Were you aware of how it felt when someone did not focus on what you were saying? You will begin to see communication in a new light.

It's worth your time and effort to shift some habits. Listening and speaking are at the top of the list. Others' habits that you find annoying are just that—annoying, not harmful. There is a marked difference and as you become tolerant of another's quirks, you might begin to find them endearing . . . or not. We all have them, but they are only part of our personalities. Try shifting your focus to the other 95 percent that you appreciate. You will be surprised at how much better life will be. As the French say, "Viva la difference!"

WEEK TWENTY-EIGHT

WORRY OR GRACE

I recently taught a program on anxiety, stress, and pain. In our discussion, one student stated that she was worried about the fact that she was worried. At first, the group found this amusing, but her insightful observation indicated that she was aware that her worry was detrimental to her physical and emotional health.

Worry affects everyone, and I am sure we could all make lists a mile long about our concerns. I find it interesting that although we know worry has no positive influence on the outcome, we still worry. For some, worry is actually an addiction—it seems to help us feel in control. We get used to it, and it undermines our enjoyment of life.

Our thoughts are exhausting and we agonize over everything. There are different opinions of how many thoughts we have per day, but the average is around 55,000. I can assure you, most of them are not uplifting! Here is an example of the process. Let's say you are planning a party. Your worry track might go like this:

> Will the party go as planned? What if someone doesn't eat meat—will the vegetables be enough or should I make something special? If I do that, will others want it and there won't be enough of that? What will happen if it rains? (This is a concern even though the gathering is inside!) One of my plates is chipped—should I use it anyway or use one that does not quite match—hmmm, what will everyone think? How can I wear this outfit again after some of my guests saw me wear it a few months ago? Oh no, two of the people I invited do not get along so I have to remember to find a way to keep them apart. What if they cancel at the last minute? What will I do with all of the leftovers?

Yes, sad but true, this is the exhausting life of worry which will continue throughout the party and, before you know it, the evening is over. You have spent tremendous effort, time, and money to be with your company and in your worry and anxiety you forgot to enjoy yourself and those around you.

We not only worry when hosting an event, but also with each and every plan and person with whom we are involved. Worry envelops us and it spills out into our relationships. "What will happen if my two-year-old doesn't get into the best preschool? I know it will affect his/her growth and future college options!" I enjoyed the perspective of comedian Tina Fey in her book *Bossypants*: "My ability to turn good news into anxiety is rivaled only by my ability to turn anxiety into chin acne." Yes, worry has a definite spiral, right down to our complexions!

Some situations are more serious, such as an illness or a financial issue, and you might be wondering how I expect you to stop worrying about them. I don't; but when you understand the consequence of worry you will realize that no matter what you are facing in life, worry will make it worse. This epidemic not only affects adults, but children as well.

The Atlanta Journal Constitution (August 8, 2011) published a feature article on the rising stress symptoms seen in children of all ages. The article, "Child Anxiety Can Be a Big Issue: Fears and Worry Seen in Kids Today" highlighted the need for psychologists to pay serious attention to symptoms of anxiety, such as panic attacks and other physical and emotional consequences. Some of the mindfulness-based stress-reduction techniques, as illustrated in Week Twenty Two are being implemented to help children see clearly what is happening in the present. They learn techniques to divert emotional reaction. The practices include breath, movement, activities, touching, tasting, smelling, seeing, and listening.

The medical community is advocating mindfully-based stress-reduction techniques to help a multitude of conditions caused by anxiety and worry. When we worry, our mind is either in the future or the past, not where we are at the moment. No matter which technique is implemented, the goal is to anchor the mind back to the here and now.

Let me divert to some philosophy that can shed some light on the subject.

In his book, *The Sacred Art of Lovingkindness*, Rabbi Rami Shapiro says that all that matters is this moment and how you engage it. There are two ways to engage this moment: with grace or with worry. He goes on to say that the opposite of grace is your own anxiety.

Grace can be thought of as effortless movement, form, or proportion. If you have watched a ballet, you will notice the movements flow with an ease that is mesmerizing. You feel relaxed, while being fully engaged in the beauty before you. No need to be concerned, you can embody grace without being graceful in movement.

On the other hand, anxiety encompasses a state of uneasiness and apprehension, and much if it stems from future uncertainties. This is paramount in every area of your life, including your livelihood.

We have looked at many tools throughout the months to help you come back to the present moment. When you apply them, you open the door for grace. Concern and anxiety are now replaced with ease and calm.

There is a prayer that can be effective when struggling with worry—The Serenity Prayer. *The New York Times* (July 11, 2008) ran an article by Laurie Goodstein concerning the disagreements over the prayer's origin. (I find this quite amusing and on point; even the Serenity Prayer is creating anxiety!) Give it a try the next time you feel worried:

> *God grant me the serenity to accept the things*
> *I cannot change, courage to change the things I can,*
> *and wisdom to know the difference.*

If you do not relate to the word God, feel free to change it to something you are comfortable with, or simply omit it.

This prayer is the embodiment of living life in the moment in all of your activities. Since you cannot change the outcome of situations, all you can do is the legwork needed and then let go of the results. They are simply not under your control.

You cannot think your way out of worrying, but what you can do is replace it with the Serenity Prayer. It is the antidote for anxiety and concern every time you say it. You will feel lighter, calmer, and have a life filled with grace when you abide by its principles.

Let's go back to the worry track I was previously discussed. Imagine your party was a complete success; you showed up in last year's outfit, in the rain, and you didn't worry about a thing. In fact, you were present to enjoy every moment. Now, *that's* living in grace. What an exquisite way to live.

AUGUST

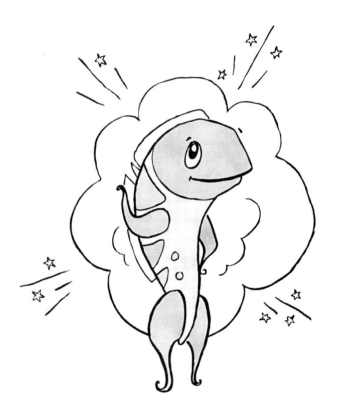

Perspective

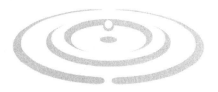

C U S T O M   C A L M

WEEK TWENTY-NINE

INTUITION AND MEDITATION

Albert Einstein's words are a great introduction to this week's entry: "No problem can be solved from the same consciousness that created it."

Consciousness can be thought of as the relationship between our mind and the world with which it interacts. Other words used to describe it are subjectivity, awareness, ability to feel, and being awake.

When we are challenged to solve problems, we focus on figuring out a solution. In our effort to do this we end up producing even more confusion, which spirals into frustration. We are unable to be objective or aware when our minds are cluttered with the same old thoughts and perceptions. We literally think our way to exhaustion, losing our ability to see new possibilities. We remain stuck in the problem. What is needed is a change in perspective.

When you look at the ocean, the first thing you notice are the waves, because they are the most visible. At times the momentum of the waves is so tumultuous that only the whitecaps can be seen. Think of the ocean's waves as thought-waves. At times your thoughts are turbulent and at other times your thoughts are calm and focused. When your mind latches onto figuring out a solution, it can get stuck in thought-waves, obscuring other possibilities.

Beneath the waves there is the vastness of the entire ocean and that is where you will find answers. The mind is only a part of who you are, but when you get stuck there, you are missing out on utilizing your full capacity. You must dive deeper to find what lies within.

We have the ability to reach deeper into our inner resources. Einstein knew that his mind and perspective had to shift to solve a problem. The evidence of what he achieved is a powerful testimony. We have to wonder how he was able to make the shift from trying to solve a problem to coming up with a solution. He took meditation naps during his working day to develop new theories. He said: "The really valuable thing is intuition," and "Through meditation I found answers before I even asked the question."

There are two areas to explore: Intuition and Meditation.

Intuition

Intuition is the ability to acquire knowledge that is beyond the use of reason. (Don't worry, I am not asking you to all be psychics.) The word "intuition" comes from the Latin word *intueri*, which is translated as "look inside or contemplate." The intuition I am highlighting is looking inside for answers. Let's think about what "inside" intuition means.

"Simple being" is a term used in many arenas. Simple being is the part of you that has always been there and will remain constant as long as you live. Throughout your life, you have changed. Your thoughts, feelings, body, tastes, environment, and relationships have all changed, but there is something within that is constant. It is a stillness that we immerse into when we are in the present moment—beyond our thought-waves.

We live in a world where we value the mind. I agree that our minds are vital to a full life, but we are so much more. We must go within—beneath the waves—to see how vast the ocean is. We have a capacity to tap into wisdom that we possess, and that is our intuition.

Meditation

I find it amusing that several times when teaching I have tripped up on the word "meditation" and said "medication" instead. Yes, one simple consonant separates the two, but I think there is something to my error. We will probably have less need for medication when we practice meditation!

We have already ascertained that when we quiet our minds we are able to stop the vicious cycle of confusion. This is why meditation practices are of great value. We need a clean slate to work with or we end up with a disorganized mess.

Rest assured, to meditate you don't have to sit in a strange position and dip into the cosmos! There are many meditation techniques to choose from to meet your specific personality needs. If you are not one to get still, then a moving meditation will work more effectively. If you love nature, then you can meditate through nature. The moment we try to quiet the mind, we realize just how busy it is. Yoga calls this the "monkey mind" because our thoughts swing from branch to branch.

One of the many reasons to meditate is to relax the body and settle the mind. Think of your mind as a jar full of liquid. If you keep pouring in more, it will overflow, making a big mess. It is necessary to first clear your thoughts so you have an empty vessel to gain a fresh perspective.

When you are having computer problems and are not sure how to fix them (you have already yelled at it and are ready to throw it out the window!), what is the first thing you try? You reboot it. Think of meditation as a reboot for your mind. For the purpose of problem-solving, just a few moments of clearing your mind will go a long way to make the shift needed to get into the solution.

Next time you are unable to solve a problem, meditate using one of the breathing practices explained in previous weeks. Many other techniques are also scattered throughout this book.

- February: Basic Breath Awareness
- May: Alternate Nostril Breathing
- June: Three Part Breath

Other objects of attention beside the breath are also effective gateways into meditation. Understand that whatever tool you use, its purpose is to give your mind a focal point on which to concentrate.

Here are a few tips:

- If possible, sit upright to meditate, either on a cushion on the floor or in a chair—whatever is most comfortable. If you need to use a different position, do so.
- Stick with one centering technique at a time; the mind will want to complicate things.
- It is natural that your mind will drift and when that happens, notice what is on your mind and gently guide it back to the tool you are using.
- If it feels like you fell asleep, you might have been experiencing inner stillness or what Einstein calls "a meditation nap." If you were indeed asleep, realize that you might simply be tired.
- Be consistent in sitting for a few minutes each day, so when you really need help with problem-solving, you will have the experience to quickly quiet your mind. Practice daily and work your way up to five minutes. (Twice a day would be even better!)

Get in the habit of meditating daily and begin to notice your state of mind. Are you calmer? Are you clearer? Remember, the point is to make space in your mind so you can see the world with more clarity. Keep practicing, even if you do not think it is helping—Einstein and I promise it will!

WEEK THIRTY

FREEDOM TO CHOOSE

Viktor Frankl spent three years in various concentration camps during World War II. He lived in an environment where every freedom was taken away and his circumstances were unimaginable, yet he knew he had a choice about what his attitude would be. We can all learn from his message: "Everything can be taken from a man or a woman but one thing: the last of human freedoms to choose one's attitude in any given set of circumstances, to choose one's own way."

I highlight Viktor Frankl as an extraordinary example of how we, as human beings, can choose how we want to view our situation and when we exercise that choice it has a significant impact on our day-to-day physical and emotional wellbeing.

Our lives are filled with situations that do not go as planned. Most of these unwanted interruptions are more of an inconvenience than a life-threatening problem, yet we often react with anger and frustration. Let's look at why this happens.

The mundane story below illustrates how even a small inconvenience still needed a shift in perspective. It shows that no matter what happens to us our attitude is the key to enjoying life.

> It was a lovely spring day, so I took some well-deserved time off. I made lunch with the intention of eating outdoors so I could enjoy the wonderful weather. I walked out to my patio with a plate filled with colorful, fragrant food and I was ready to dig in. As I was sitting down, I felt something wet drop on my head. I hoped it was some kind of leaf, but sure enough, it was bird poop!

I have heard that when bird poop lands on your head it is a sign of good luck so I investigated this claim further. Many believe this incident be a major sign of wealth coming from heaven. It is quite unpleasant and inconvenient, but when something like this happens to you take comfort in the fact that others describe it as a sign that good luck is just around the corner! (I hope this luck excludes more bird poop!)

This is a matter of perspective. At first I did not feel very lucky. After all, I had my plan in place and was treating myself to a pleasurable dining experience. I felt my mood shift to one of frustration at the inconvenience, so I made a decision to employ a centering technique in order to adjust my outlook.

My perspective made the difference in how I experienced the moments after this happened. If I had taken it as a personal affront that the bird went out of its way to find my head to poop on (the thought initially crossed my mind), I would have stayed angry from the mess in my hair and on my hand. Instead I was able to smile, clean myself off, and sit down to a wonderful lunch.

Let's look at two arenas where perspective plays a huge role:

Home Life

You might wonder how it is possible that events do not determine the quality of our day. Of course our days are influenced by events, but it's what we do about it that makes the difference. Think about how many times your day has been derailed by your attitude. It might have been the kids, behavior, traffic, or any other part of the day. Quite often, you cannot even remember what upset you.

There are days where you are just in a funky mood and your attitude exudes negativity. Perhaps you have had occasions where something occurred that has tripped an attitude change in an instant. That is lovingly known as a mood swing. Rest assured you are human so it is bound to happen from time to time.

I know that my day is determined by my perspective, not the actual events. Two people will see the same situation quite differently and we have opportunities every day to decide what our attitude will be. How you exercise this choice has a profound effect on your mental, physical, and emotional states. When we are aware that we perceive events with a negative spin, we can take a moment to get centered (use any of the techniques outlined in this book), and look at it for what it is. You will be amazed at the difference it will make in your day.

Work

I hear many people talk about working at jobs they do not enjoy but are financially unable to leave. They feel stuck, and their unhappiness results in negative attitudes and outlooks toward life. This causes stress and clouds their ability to enjoy their day. What can we do if quitting is not an option?

Oprah Winfrey said: "The greatest discovery of all time is that a person can change his future by merely changing his attitude." And I agree.

I read an article about positive thinking written by doctors at The Mayo Clinic. The overall message was: Your thoughts affect your reality, which in turn can compromise your health and well-being. (This is probably not news to any of you!) The article goes on to speak about self-talk, which is nothing more than the thoughts in the mind. I have spoken in depth about this topic. The article says the following:

> Positive thinking doesn't mean that you keep your head in the sand and ignore life's less pleasant situations. Positive thinking just means that you approach the unpleasantness in a more positive and productive way. You think the best is going to happen, not the worst....

Positive thinking often starts with self-talk. Self-talk is the endless stream of unspoken thoughts that run through your head every day.

The Mayo Clinic article cites many health benefits of having a positive attitude, which we have touched on throughout the book. Among them are:

- Increased life span
- Lower rates of depression
- Lower levels of distress

There are thousands more articles on the subject. I have included this in the work section because we sometimes need some help with living life to the fullest while being in a job that is not satisfying. Even if you enjoy your job, there is always room for an attitude adjustment.

Suze Orman, an internationally-acclaimed personal finance expert, talks about some of the financial considerations to help people decide about job change. What intrigued me was the title, the introduction, and first tip:

Change Your Attitude Before Changing Your Job. "If you are unhappy in your current job, my advice is to take a step back and see how you might be able to make it work for you. The truth that you must face is that in this lousy job market, the job you have is a great job because it is a job. You cannot afford to walk away from any job today without having another job lined up."

One item on her Mini Action Plan Reality Check was: "Your thoughts create reality, so change your attitude to make your job work for you."

It is clear, whether at work or at home, your attitude, rather than the actual events, determines your day, Begin this week to practice shifting to a more positive perspective. Start with something mundane, and remember that not everything is a big problem until you make it so. It is a process, so you will catch yourself in negativity from time to time. Some of your outlooks have been with you for years (and years and years...) and it takes time to make incremental changes.

You have the freedom to choose how you want to live your life every moment. Take a pause to readjust your attitude and then go out and enjoy your day.

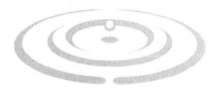

CUSTOM CALM

WEEK THIRTY-ONE

ATTITUDE OF GRATITUDE

There is a saying (and now the title of a popular song): "What doesn't kill you will make you stronger." I am sure you would find it hard to use those words while going through a challenging situation, but at some point it is possible.

I find it interesting that so many of the most inspiring people in the world had to endure major hurdles. Helen Keller had unimaginable obstacles to overcome in her life and she said: "I thank God for my handicaps, for through them I have found myself, my work, and my God."

She had so many limitations that to cultivate a purposeful and fulfilling life, she needed to look within for strength and fortitude. Think about those in your life who have had a positive influence on you. You will find they developed into who they are because of their life experiences, not in spite of them. We are all shaped by events we have participated in and every day we continue to have new encounters, but it is our nature to only accept the happy, uplifting situations.

In daily living, we feel overwhelmed when things do not go as planned. It is during this time that gratitude helps to soften what seems never ending. The challenge is finding gratitude in the midst of frustration, fear, and uncertainty.

When I look back at what I considered to be my most difficult times, I realize that those events propelled me to change and grow. I feel safe to say that much of this book has come as a result of those experiences. We all have our stories, but some continue to stay stuck and perpetuate negative feelings.

We looked at positive thinking last week. Gratitude is another attitude that facilitates positive thinking. We touched on it back in February, and now we will examine it a bit more. Having gratitude for the difficult times is not easy for many of us to understand. We tend to focus on the struggle, hurt, and pain that we encountered, so why should we be grateful?

This brings to mind a conversation with an elder I once taught. He told me that he was often thinking about past events that impacted his life. He told me a few stories and they were all about wrongs that he felt were done to him. He was wallowing in these memories and, I am told, lived much of his life speaking about them.

I watched this man who has lived a wonderful, long, fulfilling life surrounded by friends and family who love him. And yet his focus was on the negative events. I joked with him and asked, "If it was painful when it happened years back, why would you want to continue to relive the experience over and over again? It wasn't fun the first time!" I might have been joking, but it holds great truth.

We all have encountered unpleasant situations and we seem to remember them in detail. Our negative experiences stem from either something that was done to us, something that we did, or something that we had no control over. When we continue to relive the negative, we perpetuate whatever feelings we had, bringing them into the present day. What stems from our minds, rather than the actual past events, creates our reality.

It is helpful to review what happened so you can gain some insight. Some questions to ask might be: "What could I have done differently?" and "Is there another way to look at the situation?" While reviewing an experience, don't neglect the fact that there might have been some uplifting moments as well, no matter how insignificant. While the sweet, small events we engaged in are often overshadowed by our upsetting memories, make sure you include them in your review, and then move forward. Even forgiveness is a choice.

Gratitude is the antidote for day-to-day annoyances as well as difficult times. You do not have to *feel* grateful to *be* grateful. To begin with, you can "act as if" you are grateful and that alone will make a shift. Gratitude is a decision and it is your choice. When you live in gratitude, it will ripple over into your relationships and experiences, helping you to fully participate in daily life.

The question is: How to transform our mindset when we are conditioned to think in a certain way? How do we accomplish this shift in perspective? It's the glass half-empty/half-full scenario, and our perspective will make a big difference.

Try this when you are up against something you do not want to do:

- Next time you are annoyed at paying bills or preparing your taxes, take a breath and think about how blessed you are to have the income and ability to pay bills. This is a good problem to have!

Try this when you are feeling negative or overwhelmed and find yourself complaining:

- Take a slow easy breath... and another one.
- Feel your feet on the floor.
- Bring to mind some experience that you found enjoyable, no matter how insignificant.
- While taking a few more breaths, stay focused on the feelings it evoked.
- With each slow, deep inhalation and exhalation, say the words "Thank You."
- If that does not work for you, go back to Week Thirteen in April and try the smile breath.

Try this when there a major obstacle to overcome or if you are feeling negative about yourself:

- Take a slow easy breath... and another one.
- Feel your feet on the floor.
- Take a moment and bring to mind some small challenge that you have gone through. If you cannot think of one, bring to mind someone in your life who has faced a challenge.
- Look for one small positive outcome—maybe it shaped your perceptions, activities, spiritual path, or relationships.
- While you do this, keep this saying in mind: "Keep digging, there's got to be a pony under this pile of %?#@? somewhere!" (Even if you cannot overcome the obstacle, the image in itself should make you smile and will help you make the shift.)

Keep in mind that everything takes time. Those who have been role models did not feel or behave with gratitude while they were going through the struggle, but it came in hindsight. In their choice to move forward through adversity, they developed an unshakable inner knowing right down to their core. Life is not intended to be a struggle. You have the capacity and choice to see your experiences differently. Why not use them?

WEEK THIRTY-TWO

THAT'S LIFE: JAMIE'S STORY

At this juncture, I'd like to share an excerpt from a paper written by my younger daughter. When she was eight, she was diagnosed with an uncommon form of muscular dystrophy. I am sharing a story she wrote eight years later because it is a powerful example of how one's perspective can make a difference.

Her assignment was to write a story about an event that shaped her life in some way. She picked her illness and wrote the story as if it was a script for a play, in her voice. I need to tell you, no one helped her with this.

Jamie as a young adult reflecting back
It's amazing to me how I ever survived. I have been sick with a disease for 11 years now. The disease is called dermatomyositis. Don't worry about pronouncing it; hopefully, you'll never need to. I wondered why this was happening to me, and I wished I had never gotten sick... It never occurred to me until later on that everything really does happen for a reason.

Set: Softball field, Jamie is at bat, she is eight years old, and about to turn nine.

The crowd cheers as Jamie hits the ball to the infield.

Mom: She isn't hitting as well as she used to. She is running slowly now, too. I'm getting worried, Robert.

Dad: I'm sure it's nothing, Ellen. She probably just needs practice.

Umpire: OUT!

Sister (jokingly): Next time you might want to try running instead of jogging, Jamie.

Jamie: I was running as fast as I could, okay!?

At the table, after her older sister gets frustrated with her whining

Jamie Thinking: She thought I was faking. I wasn't. I wish I were just faking. My parents couldn't figure out what was wrong with me. The doctors couldn't even figure out what was wrong with me. I couldn't even figure out what was wrong with me! You know how you have kind of like a sixth sense where you know that something is going wrong. Well, about this time my sixth sense was going haywire. I even got so sick I couldn't tie my shoes or lift my head off the pillow. Finally, a dear friend (doctor) of ours had an idea of what was wrong with me. She said I might have dermatomyositis. She said she couldn't do anything but she would get us an appointment with a doctor. (Well, test after test went by, and it was dermatomyositis.) I remember the first test I went to. The doctor was wearing a tie-dye shirt, and he gave me a lion stuffed animal with a little heart necklace. He said it was for courage. Now I know how much I needed it . . . .

You never realize how many people care about you. I remember that every time I went to the hospital, at least three friends would visit. I remember getting cards, and phone calls, and presents. It makes you feel so good. I can't imagine what going to the hospital would be like without all those people who care. Not just people came for me, but they came for my mom when she was in the hospital with me. It makes you want to just cry. I remember when I went to the Mayo Clinic. In the hotel room, I got calls and faxes from all of my friends, and when I got back home, everyone came to visit me . . . . I remember when they gave me that stupid back brace. I remember those trips to Chicago to see the doctor who treated me more as a guinea pig than a patient. Those were the times where I wished most that I wasn't in that situation. But, as I said before, everything happens for a reason, even if you don't see it right away.

Dressing Room – Jamie is getting her hair ready
She is very excited because she is about to be on TV (She was the ambassador for the Georgia Muscular Dystrophy Association (MDA)). As she is preparing she is thinking about what she will say.

Jamie – Standing in front of the mirror in a hotel room, she is talking to herself
Okay . . . one last time. Interviewer: Why should those people donate to MDA? Me: Well, MDA does so many things for people with muscular dystrophy. They send kids to camp, have free clinic visits, provide leg braces and wheel chairs. They do everything. Interviewer: Wow! That is a lot of stuff, and it's all free? Me: Yup. And every year they hold other amazing fund-raisers. So even if you can't donate this time, please, try next time. Interviewer: Thanks, Jamie. Me: No problem.

(She smiles) I can't wait until I get interviewed. [Jamie raised over $8,000 that year.]

Here is her last paragraph
It's true, I was finally getting better. After five long, miserable years I was finally getting better. Actually, I wouldn't quite call them miserable. They were bad, but I can't help but have this feeling about those years. I know this sounds crazy, but if I could choose to get sick or not, I don't know that I would have chosen not to have the illness. True, this disease has been a horrible thing, but I would not be the person I am today without it. It has given me a sense of compassion for everyone. It has taught me not to take simple things like walking for granted. I also can't imagine life without the people I met because of my disease. With this disease came great loss, but loss does not come with-

out gain. Every time you lose something, whether it is a loved one, or just a toy, you learn something. My disease is part of who I am. I am proud of who I am, and wouldn't change it for the world. So, I guess I have a sense of why this happened to me. Because you know, everything happens for a reason. That's life.

As I read what my daughter wrote, there is really nothing I can add. She says it all. My husband, my children, and my extended family were shaped by her experience of pain and illness. We all have our lessons to learn and we watched Jamie choose a positive perspective on her circumstances. Jennifer, her older sister, suddenly had to take a back seat as the focus shifted to her sister. I am forever grateful for Jennifer's patience (most of the time) and her ability to be adaptable. It was not easy, but we all took Jamie's lead as we watched her enjoy and cultivate her activities and interests.

Today, Jamie is healthy and continues to embrace life each day. Her illness shaped us all and we came though it with a deeper awareness of what is important in life. Jamie's story illustrates how we cannot always choose what happens to us, but we can choose how we want to live. And yes, *that's life*...

SEPTEMBER

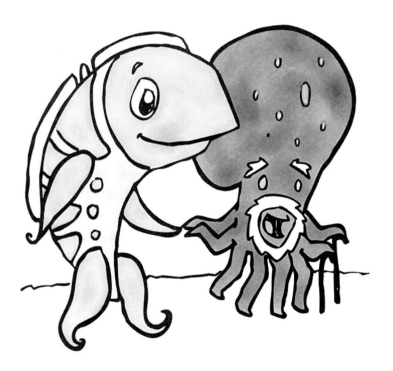

Responsibility

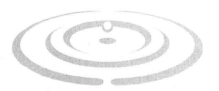

CUSTOM CALM

WEEK THIRTY-THREE

SELF CARE

Recently, my husband and I took a well needed retreat at an isolated bed and breakfast. It was a cozy, lovely facility with great food, massages, and other amenities to choose from.

A single woman showed up late the first evening, looking quite harried and stressed. She had gotten a late start and drove through the rain. While chatting, she informed me that she made a last-minute decision to leave her children home with a sitter and take the weekend for herself (a stroke of genius). This was new to her and as the weekend progressed, I watched her unwind and relax so much that she did not know how to deal with her state of mind. It was as if her mind, which was on constant vigilance, could finally let go. (I think we call this a return to sanity.)

After a massage I watched her sashay down the hallway with a grin on her face. (It was good it was a wide hallway because she was weaving.) This was her first massage and I feel safe to say, not her last.

She had never taken a full weekend off to let go of her responsibilities as a single mom and full-time employee. She told me the reason she was late was because she had been in the emergency room because of a flair-up of a medical condition which was exacerbated by stress. The pampering she received gave her both the physical and emotional relief she needed.

It was a pleasure to watch her smile, take her time, and enjoy the easy, quiet pace. Having responsibilities as a mom and employee, she neglected herself. She was grateful that she had decided to leave her children home rather than bring them, since she knew she would have had to entertain them and make sure they did not disturb the other visitors. (Not a good vacation idea.) The important point to understand is that if we don't take breaks in our week for relaxation, then our well-being is compromised.

I was pondering the question, "What prevents us from taking time away from children, even when there are competent options for child care?" The problem stems from the fact that we do not think anyone beside ourselves is capable of properly looking after our cherished offspring. I admit that when my children were young, I fit into that category. For me to leave for an evening with friends meant my husband had to bathe and feed our children. My fear of returning to poor, dirty, starving waifs was never realized. Of course, in my mind, he could not do it as well as me, but somehow they survived and probably prospered despite eating unhealthy treats and having a great time.

When we finally give ourselves permission to go out with our significant other or friends, we are either on the phone every fifteen minutes checking on the children or the entire conversation is about our children. When we do this, are we really nourishing ourselves through the enjoyment and camaraderie of being with others? Are we giving ourselves permission to relinquish our responsibilities for a short time? Even a car must be refueled and maintained to operate efficiently.

It is always amusing when I hear the rules and regulations that grandparents are given when watching their grandchildren. The fact that they raised one or more of their own is not considered when evaluating their ability to babysit. (Or maybe we realize how messed up we are and do not want to perpetuate this to yet another generation)

If you cannot relate because you do not have children, do not feel left out. Replace the word children with work, any other person, place, and thing that you place before your own well-being.

When I suggest that someone take the time to "fill-up" I get the response: "Taking time to pamper myself is a luxury that I do not have." The irony is that when you take care of yourself, you will have more time and energy for your other responsibilities.

So, how do we fill-up when there is only so much time in the day?

Breathing

It seems silly to place so much emphasis on breathing because it happens naturally! But it truly opens the door to physical and emotional health. Breath oxygenates and relaxes the body, while quieting the mind. It is the least expensive, quickest way to improve your overall well-being.

Despite its simplicity and life-changing benefits, you often hold your breath. With this simple trick, you will remember to actively breathe throughout the day. Take sticky notes or index cards, and write one word in bold: **Breathe**. Stick them to your mirror where you brush your teeth, your refrigerator, your car, your desk, and anywhere else you want. (I put one on my dashboard which was a great conversation piece for my passengers.) This might seem a bit simplistic, but it is quite effective. You will be amazed what a simple reminder can do.

Relaxation Pose

Yes, there is a pose for relaxation and yoga calls it *Shavasana*. It invites us to let go completely and rest in awareness of the moment while fostering a deep sense of relaxation. It is a resting pose for both body and mind.

Try this:

- Lie on your back with your legs propped over a chair or blankets, or simply bend your knees and keep your feet on the floor—this support is effective in releasing pressure on the lumbar spine.
- Prop your head so your forehead is level with your chin—you do not want your head to tilt back as this causes neck compression.

- Allow your arms to rest near your sides with your palms facing up, or you can bend your elbows and place your hands on your belly.
- If your mind is busy, place a few folded blankets on your chest. (I had a student who finally relaxed after piling on six.)
- Rest here for 5-10 minutes with easy breathing, as you allow your body to sink heavier into the surface beneath you.

These simple practices will fortify your ability to respond effectively throughout your day. Think about it: a small investment of a few minutes will generate tremendous gains. It is a win-win for you and every other person, place, and thing you are committed to. For those with children or other commitments, an evening out will go a long way; so take care and have some adult time. You have earned it!

WEEK THIRTY-FOUR

HEALTH CHALLENGES OF LOVED ONES

In years past, I taught a one-hour monthly class at the Bone Marrow Transplant Unit at Northside Hospital to help caregivers lower stress and pain. These family members would sit for hours and days while their loved ones received infusions. Class attendance was very low and after unsuccessfully trying to motivate caregivers to participate, the program was canceled. Although they had traveled far to get to the center, the caregivers, it seemed, wouldn't even travel across the hall for an hour of self-nurturance. This is the reality of caring for loved ones and it is easy for caregivers to neglect themselves. What can we do to help them take personal care?

While flying home after a visit out of state, I picked up the June 2011 issue of *Sky Magazine*. It cited the intervention of CEOs on the devastating effects of cancer. The workplace is now included in the battle to reduce cancer's impact as well as other illnesses. This information was part of an article: "The Responsibility of Helping with Illness Goes Far Beyond the Family." It stated, "Many corporations are paying incentives for employees to participate in healthy living programs. Studies were done on participating employees and the overall health improved dramatically."

Patrick Geraghty, President and CEO of Blue Cross and Blue Shield of Florida, stated: "We have to make wellness something that businesses are focused on, because we spend so much time in the workplace." It is clear that serious illness affects us all and corporations are losing billions of dollars because if it.

When you travel by plane (as long as I have sidetracked into travel), one of the first instructions you are given is to put the oxygen mask on yourself first before putting it on the person next to you. Of course our natural instinct is to want to quickly assist our loved one, but if we do not help ourselves first, our ability to support others is compromised.

When you see the evidence of the impact that stress has on family members and caregivers, you will take it quite seriously. I will go into stress more thoroughly in the month of December, but for now, we will continue to look at the impact of chronic illness—everything from a life threatening illness, arthritis, fibromyalgia, and disabilities to ADHD. Let me begin with my own caregiver experience.

Years back, my daughter had a chronic and quite uncommon illness. One day I received a call from a young woman, Susan. Somehow my mother (leave it to a mother) ran into a friend who knew someone who dealt with the same illness and passed along my number. This young woman said something that has stuck with me throughout the years. She told me that during the years she was ill, her mother totally focused on her illness, neglecting herself.

This might sound totally appropriate, but keep an open mind as you read on. When Susan began to recover and went off to graduate school, her mother resented her. She told me that her mother felt lost without caretaking and did not know how to live her life. Susan believed that she had abandoned her mother, and felt pain and guilt. After that call I made a decision not to follow in her mother's footsteps. I could see how my identity had become tied to my role as a caregiver and that seemed to be my entire focus. I never heard from the young woman again, but am eternally grateful to her.

It is appropriate now to briefly recap a yoga teaching I spoke of in Week Thirty-Three. It tells us that we are all so much more than our bodies and identities. Whether our loved one improves or not, we must remember as their life goes by, so does ours. When we fill our tank, we can give from a space of love and compassion rather than exhaustion and worry.

Love

This brings me to the topic of love (I promise I will not get corny). Many equate love with being worried or entirely revolving your life around another. People around us might see us as being unloving and selfish if our loved feels sick and we still find time to enjoy ourselves. To me, this is love. How can we better teach family members to take care of themselves than by modeling it?

I realize that part of my path was to raise a chronically-ill child along with her healthy sibling; yet my children, my husband, and I (and I can't leave out the dog) are so much more than that. When I can remember this, I am able to balance my responsibility and love for my family with self-love and nurturance. There are many areas in life where we are loved and needed but most importantly we must be responsible to ourselves. My journey with Jamie led me to a fulfilling vocation to help others with pain, stress, and chronic illness, and I love that I am able to guide them to a place of acceptance, healing and empowerment.

Powerlessness

Recently, I have spoken with many who are ill or are caring for a sick loved one. My work at the cancer center provides many opportunities to hear stories from caretakers; I see one common thread woven throughout—they deeply care, love, and want the best for the one who is struggling.

Both the caregiver and the person who is ill undergo physical or emotional pain. They feel responsible to one another, wanting to fix the situation. They try to get the other to understand that there are things they can do to help themselves, but to no avail. We wonder why they will not do what we suggest and are certain if they did, it would help them. (This happens in every relationship.) This leads to frustration, fear, hurt, and anger. The one thing we need to remember is that we are absolutely *powerless* over the other person.

It is their life and their path; nothing we do or say will change them. This resistance is difficult for many to understand, but all we can do is to remember that we are powerless and once we realize this, we can let go of what we think they should do, lighten up, and meet them where they are.

Your shift in attitude will empower you and your relationships. You will be able to spend your energy taking care of yourself in a way that nourishes you and others. Think of all the suggestions in this and other weeks as your oxygen mask, so you may give your loved ones the gift of self-love.

WEEK THIRTY-FIVE

CAREGIVING FOR ELDERS

The following quotes focusing on caring for elders illustrates the range of problems challenging many families.

"People are living longer, and with chronic disease. Somebody's got to take care of them, and it's us," says Gail Hunt, Chief Executive Officer of the National Alliance for Caregiving.

The Baby Boomer generation (of which I am a proud member) is facing many challenges inherent in caregiving for their elder family members. Caregiving for elders affects families, health, finances, businesses, and relationships, and the need for it has become an epidemic.

The following June 4, 2011, *Wall Street Journal* article addresses this concern:

> A steep rise in people caring for elderly parents is taking a toll on the health and finances of many baby boomers, a new study says....
>
> Older caregivers who work and provide care to a parent at the same time are more likely than other workers in their age group to report poor health, with problems including depression and chronic disease. There is evidence they "experience considerable health issues as a result of their focus on caring for others," the report says.

Another study released last year by MetLife and the National Alliance for Caregiving found that depression, hypertension, diabetes, and pulmonary disease were among caregivers' more common health problems. They also experienced higher rates of stress, were more likely to smoke or drink alcoholic beverages, and were less likely to get preventive health screenings, including mammograms.

An *Atlanta Journal Constitution* article on The Alzheimer's Generation is titled: "Caregiver's Anguish: I need to be 2 people," focuses on the anguish of double-duty caregiving for the sick parent and their children—the plight of the middle-aged "sandwich generation."

I can cite thousands of articles on the topic of caregiving for elders, but the examples above illustrate my point. There is no easy answer to this problem, so we tend to get stuck in the problem. What we need is some sort of shift to help us move into the solution.

Compassion

Elders are often stuck in their way of thinking (they are not the only ones) and communication can be quite frustrating. It is clear that no matter what is said, they are not going to change. We try anyway, exacerbating tension and frustration on both sides.

It is easy to practice compassion when you are not so invested in the situation, but the challenge is to practice compassion in a relationship in which you care deeply. The best example is the parent who "pushes your buttons." You may remember we talked about this in Week Twenty Five, and I would recommend that you re-read some of the entries in February to go deeper into compassion. It is an important element in dealing with elders.

My parents are in their 90s. (Everyone says what great genes I have and I shake my head and reply, "I'm not so sure—I'm adopted!") Communicating with my parents is difficult when I get caught up in arguing and judging their perceptions and feelings—this costs us all. We become so focused on making our point, we lose sight of the love we have for one another.

I attended a program (which was packed) presented by Jewish Family Career Services in Atlanta on caregiving for elders. They recommended that we meet our elders where they are. What your elder is telling you is their reality and to argue is futile, yet we do it anyway. Here is the most difficult challenge—even if you know you are correct, agree with them anyway. It will help you avoid unnecessary tension. In Week Twenty-Six, I asked the question, "Would you rather be right, or would you rather be happy?" You do have a choice in this area: keep fighting or practice compassion.

After attending this program, I made a decision to take time to enjoy my parents and to stay away from conversations that are charged. We laugh and engage in what we enjoy talking about and when the conversation gets challenging, I shift the subject to something more neutral (the weather is my fallback).

I have found that when we see our loved ones as vulnerable human beings with fears and struggles, it is easier to remain compassionate. I invite you all to make this shift.

Filling Up

When our lives center on caring for a parent, before long we begin to neglect our own needs. We do not take time to eat properly, exercise, or participate in the activities we used to enjoy. We grow frustrated, angry, and depleted. It wreaks havoc on our immune system and we pay the consequence. We feel guilty for feeling this way when our loved one is suffering, and that perpetuates the spiral.

Remember, you cannot give what you do not have. It is vital to remember to take care of yourself, which will help everyone involved. Take a look at the suggestions below for some ideas on how to fill-up.

First, check in with yourself with this acronym: HALT. You do not want to get too Hungry, Angry, Lonely, or Tired. Any of these can take you off the beam. Use HALT to target the area in your life which has become depleted or off course.

Here are a few simple ideas to help:

- Do a few yoga stretches.
- Stand and shake your body out—it is okay if you look silly.
- Make sure to eat nutritious food even when you do not feel like it, and drink plenty of water.
- Change the book you are reading to something funny and uplifting.
- Watch an upbeat, inspiring movie. (No murder mysteries—you might get ideas!)
- Call a friend and just vent, and then talk about something uplifting.
- Find a support group that emphasizes the solution.
- Take off your shoes, go outside (keep shoes on if below 40° or icy) and feel your feet in the earth.
- Always keep a sense of humor. Look for something funny or smile even if you do not feel like it.
- If you have time, get a manicure, pedicure, or massage. (Getting all of them would really fill you up!)

Do a breathing practice. The following, simple Ocean Sounding Breath is very helpful in allowing you to relax and to give your body some well needed rest:

- Practice either lying down or sitting upright, with your chin slightly tucked.
- To find the sound, pretend you are fogging a mirror through your mouth and then do it again with your mouth closed. It is the sound that you make when you are trying to whisper to get someone's attention with no one else hearing you.

- Gently narrow the back of your throat passages and breathe in and out through your nose. The sound is similar to the sound of a conch shell at your ear, or when you submerge your ears below water. It also reminds me of the sound of Darth Vader's voice from *Star Wars*.
- Once you have the soft ocean sound, make it smooth and steady. You are breathing normally, but with a gentle narrowing at the back of your throat. The key is to listen to the sound of your breath and make it so quiet that only you can hear it, both on the inhale and exhale. Every time you have a thought (and you will), guide your awareness back to the sound of your breath. If you cannot find this sound or are staining, then listen to your easy breathing.

I realize that you have limited time to care for yourself, but when you take a few moments throughout the day to fill up, you will be able to keep the care in caregiving. Compassion and self-love are the main ingredients. Remember, you cannot care for others if you don't care for yourself.

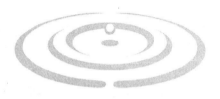

CUSTOM CALM

WEEK THIRTY-SIX

RESPONSIBILITY EQUALS FREEDOM

A friend and I were having a discussion about responsibility, and he said freedom cannot exist without responsibility. He felt that each stage of responsibility must be sustained with the proportionate amount of freedom, or problems could arise. This needs to occur at each new level of freedom. I agree with him.

Eleanor Roosevelt said: "Freedom makes a huge requirement of every human being. With freedom comes responsibility. For the person who is unwilling to grow up, the person who does not want to carry his own weight, this is a frightening prospect."

The Week Fourteen entry in April about Passover and Easter explored how our minds keep us bound, obscuring our access to the inner experience of freedom we yearn for. The previous entries this month highlighted the importance of taking care of ourselves so we can be responsible to one another. Let's take both themes a step further and look at the responsibility inherent in freedom.

The classic story by J.M. Barrie, *Peter Pan or The Boy Who Wouldn't Grow Up* has an underlying theme equating growing up with unwanted responsibility. "I Won't Grow Up," the song from the movie, is timeless, and the title alone captures our resistance to growing up and taking on added responsibility.

The added burdens and worry associated with growing up seem to be the largest deterrent to our desire to mature. To live in Neverland seems exciting and appealing, but it is a fantasy. (Sorry to burst your bubble.) Even in Neverland the characters had responsibilities. They had to protect themselves, find food, clothing, and shelter, or they would have lost the freedom to live the life they yearned for.

As parents, we try to teach this lesson to our children by assigning chores (responsibility) and rewarding them with an allowance or privileges for their participation (freedom). Responsibility carries a duty and accountability toward one's self and others. For many, however, responsibility carries a negative connotation, when it is quite the opposite—it means we now have freedom if we choose to take it. When we are free, we have the power to act or think without limits being placed upon us. We must treat this power with reverence, because without care and consideration chaos will ensue.

Let's look at a few examples at the cost of too much freedom without personal responsibility: driving while under the influence, texting while driving, tailing, and speeding are all irresponsible behaviors. Maybe we were given more freedoms with our driver's license than we were ready for. We end up getting into an accident, which can take our freedom away completely. We see this sad reality with teen drivers and the cost is high. Another example is people who become successful quickly. They come into large sums of money and either spend it recklessly, or use if for power and control. Either way, their level of responsibility was not proportionate to the freedom they gained, resulting in chaos and loss.

Since we do not live on an isolated island (though I admit there are times I have entertained this idea), our actions ripple further than we realize. Our responsibility must reach beyond ourselves, because we are all connected. It includes our relationships, our community, and our planet. This can feel quite daunting but it is essential to have a balance of responsibility and freedom.

I knew a college law professor years back who shared his frustration over an incident. He caught a group of students in his undergraduate law class cheating on exams. (I am sad to report that it was a business law class on ethics.)

He gave them consequences and in addition he required them to write a paper (Today, they would have been expelled.) on the Categorical Imperative of cheating. The Categorical Imperative, the central concept in the moral philosophy of Immanuel Kant is founded on duty-based ethics and can be used as a guide in evaluating motivations for action. In deciding whether or not an action is ethical, we should consider what the effect would be if everyone acted in the same way. The students had to write a paper in answer to the question: If everyone in the class cheated, how would that impact the class? I thought this assignment quite appropriate for teaching a lesson, because our behavior has an influence that reaches far beyond the individual.

Only when we are responsible for our behavior are we free. There is no one to blame and no resentment that ensues. In other words, the only person you can change is *you*. That simple sentence is very liberating. It takes others out of the equation and puts the responsibility for your behavior and state of mind in your hands. Even if someone wronged you, it is up to you to keep your side of the street clean, which might be as simple as a shift in attitude. There is great empowerment in living this way. No matter what happens, you are never the victim.

When I hear people ask the question, *"Why me?"* my answer is, *"Why not?"* This is the harsh truth and in no way do I want to seem heartless. When you understand that life will always have its ups and downs and you allow time to settle into the reality of a difficult experience, then you can choose how you want to perceive what has happened. There is a palpable difference between those who live with an attitude of empowerment and gratitude and those who live as a victim of their circumstances.

When you take responsibility for your mind-set and actions, you will live with greater peace of mind. Inner calm will replace fear and resistance. I want to assure you that calm does not mean boring; on the contrary, it means fully participating in the joy of living.

Remember, you have the freedom to choose what you want to focus on: the problem or the solution. When you live in solution as Eleanor Roosevelt said, you are "carrying your weight," and you will live a life that is liberating, nourishing, and exciting.

OCTOBER

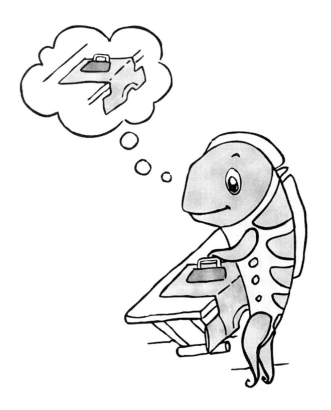

Day-to-Day Living

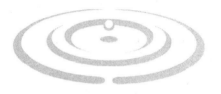

CUSTOM CALM

WEEK THIRTY-SEVEN

SIMPLE PLEASURES

This topic is important because it sheds some light on how much of our daily experiences go unnoticed. There are many reasons for this, and they all stem from our minds. Let's take a look at a few common instances where we dwell either in the past or future, causing us to miss out on what is right in front of us.

Expectation

My husband and I were on vacation out West and heard about some picturesque hiking paths. Our first hike was a mile-long trail that ended at a waterfall. What began as an easy walk soon became an uphill climb. (We now know short does not equal easy.)

As we took in the beauty around us (as well as our leg fatigue) we heard a couple behind us complaining about how difficult the path was. They kept debating whether or not to continue. As we neared the end, the couple asked us to check out the waterfall to see if it was worth finishing the trail.

It was pretty, but nothing unusual and we reported this to the couple. They decided not to continue and complained about the disappointment on their way back.

I was thinking about how they failed to see the beauty surrounding them throughout the hike, since their focus was on the difficulty of the hike and final destination. As they pushed toward the waterfall, they got trapped by the expectation of what they thought the waterfall was going to be, missing what was right in front of them.

Our thoughts produce expectations about our experience, taking us out of the here and now. At times our expectations fall short of the actual event and other times our expectations are surpassed. Either way, think about how much we miss when we focus on the future. Enjoy the journey; it is as important as the final destination.

Routines

Routines are part of our daily lives. Often, we do not notice what we are doing, as the routine is deeply ingrained in our day. The daily shower is a great example of how much more there is to experience from the simple activity of getting clean.

Have you ever taken a shower and forgot how many times you have shampooed? Maybe you have showered and you were thinking about an upcoming meeting or reviewing the list of things you had to do for the family.

Whatever you were thinking about, it kept you from enjoying the feeling of the water on your body, the warmth when you rinse the lather of shampoo out of your hair (if you are bald this still applies), or even belting out your favorite tune. You were showering alone (yes, I am making this assumption), but there was an entire committee there with you!

When you pay attention and embrace the moment you will discover how much there is to relish in your everyday routines.

Errands

Throughout the day we have our to-do list and much of it involves shopping of some kind. (Do not get excited, I am not going to talk about a shopping spree. Many of us already have mastered that kind of errand!) I am targeting our experience of mundane errands.

How much time do we spend, on a daily basis, getting our errands over with? We might rush to pick up at the cleaners, purchase something at the hardware store, or go grocery shopping, trying to accomplish as much as possible. When we live this way, we close the door to opportunities for enjoying ourselves. The mundane errands are just as much a part of life as our sports, luncheons, or vacations.

The supermarket is a great place to begin cultivating awareness of your surroundings. Give this a try next time you are at the market:

- Go to the produce aisle.
- Stand and look around; take in the total scope of what is in front of you.
- Walk around and focus on the colors, textures, shapes, and smells.
- While going down the other aisles, continue to look at the displays, colors, shapes, people you pass, and whatever else comes into view.
- Notice the sensation in your body as you do this.
- If you find you are no longer present to what you are doing, stop and take a breath.
- When checking out, look at your items as you put them on the counter.
- Look your cashier in the eye and thank them when you finish.

You will see just how much there is to take in and you will leave feeling refreshed. Think of it as a vacation at the market!

Time

I hear the term "killing time" and I wonder why anyone would want to kill time when that is life going by. We have the perception that what we are participating in is not worth our time and is simply something to get out of the way.

Often when waiting for something or someone, we have time to spare before the next activity. Many of us have endured waiting in the carpool line where signs are posted that forbid the use of cell phones (the speaker phone and earpiece help mask our resistance to this rule). We are not even allowed to leave the car to chat with another carpool hostage. Some bring books or work to do to with the intention of passing time.

You can try watching and noticing your surroundings. Even while sitting in your car you will begin to see how much is going on each moment. When we learn to get still and are at ease with waiting, we can take advantage of the opportunity to fill up and reconnect with ourselves.

All of these situations offer many possibilities to take pleasure in day-to-day living. When you live where your feet are planted you will discover the full range of what is right before your eyes. Reframe your daily routines and errands and treat them as events to participate in, rather than something to get through. Next time you think about *killing* time, remember to savor each moment, because the present moment is all you have.

WEEK THIRTY-EIGHT

HOUSEHOLD DUTIES

I was teaching a course about being mindful of everyday tasks and one of my students told me that much of his day was spent on boring household tasks such as dusting and vacuuming. He did not enjoy this but it was his responsibility, and he tried to get it over with as quickly as he could.

Let's take last week's teaching a step further and examine how the approach we take toward even the most mundane tasks influences our lives.

We all have household responsibilities that can be a bit cumbersome and unexciting. Some of them we enjoy, some we don't mind, and others we really dislike; but they all need to get accomplished.

My sister is one of those neat people and enjoys organizing and getting things clean. (We all need at least one of these people in our lives.) While she was visiting our home, I gave her the pleasure of cleaning my makeup case (actually, she grabbed it from me). I watched her carefully clean it and I must admit it looked like new when she was finished. Smears of makeup on my makeup case does not bother me so it never occured to me to clean it. However, I do not like wearing wrinkly clothes, so even my t-shirts get ironed. Some people think this is nuts, but most of the time I actually do not mind ironing. I watch the wrinkles leave as I pay attention to what is in front of me and it is quite therapeutic as it brings me to the moment. (Another advantage of being present is that I avoid burning myself or my clothing.) No matter how we feel about the task at hand, are we able to show the same care and awareness as the things we deem important?

There are times each day where we partake in some kind of mundane task, so why not allow ourselves to stay present rather than mindlessly get it over with? When we only stay present to the parts of our life that we find exciting or pleasurable, then we, and those around us, miss out on the range of possibilities to fill up, connect, and enjoy.

There is a yoga teaching that addresses the importance of being mindful even when engaged in a mundane task. In Sanskrit it says: *Lokanandah Samadhi Sukham*, which can be translated into the following:

> *In every bit of knowledge, the yogi experiences the delight of I Consciousness, and there is transmission of this experience to those who come in contact with him. The bliss continues in every location and every situation.*

Okay, so the English translation is as complex as the Sanskrit! I promise there is simplicity beyond the words. When we looked at lovingkindness in February (Week Six) I introduced this concept, and now we will dive into it a bit further.

Picture this: you just finished your centering practices and you are peaceful and content. You amble into the kitchen to join your family. The kids are yelling, the dog is barking, and your significant other is looking for the keys. Poof! Your serenity has gone out the window! Where did it go? You had it a minute ago!

This teaching tells us that the bliss is firmly grounded within, everywhere you are. Bring it with you—from your walk in the woods, the meditation room, or any other area where you feel peaceful—into everything, even your own chaotic family. You can live in a world where the bliss never leaves. Nice thought, and although it doesn't seem possible, it is.

First let's explore the meaning of bliss. Bliss can be thought of as serene joy. Can we maintain serene joy while engaged in the mundane? It is easy to get to a blissful state when you are overlooking the Grand Canyon (unless you are afraid of heights), when you look at a beautiful sunset, or when you are on retreat, but what about in your day-to-day living? What happens to our inner state when there is disarray?

Back in Week Twenty we touched on our capacity to access inner stillness and it is a key ingredient of staying anchored in happiness and joy. I am not suggesting we all go skipping around laughing all the time (that would be a bit scary), but we can experience joy that is palpable from the inside-out. This occurs when you are grounded in the present moment and steady in your own knowing. You can live this way, even when people are complaining or your boss is in a bad mood.

"Weave in the divine with the mundane," is the essence of this yoga teaching. It says you will experience "delight in I Consciousness" and that you will "transmit this experience to others." You are embodied consciousness and when you quiet your mind to become aware of the unfolding moment, you encounter this sweet state of mind. When you live this way, there is a deep awareness of who you are and it will radiate from every pore, touching everyone around you. It cannot be diminished or increased by anything external, no matter how mundane the activity.

"Live your life with grounded presence, weaving in the sublime with the mundane." It does not matter whether you are surrounded by loved ones, chaos, or the pots and pans in the kitchen, your inner knowing remains unshakable and that is the essence of living in bliss.

Eckhart Tolle, in his book *The Power of Now: A Guide to Spiritual Enlightenment* says: "As soon as you honor the present moment, all unhappiness and struggle dissolve, and life begins to flow with joy and ease. When you act out the present-moment awareness, whatever you do becomes imbued with a sense of quality, care, and love—even the most simple action."

There are simple practices that will cultivate the moment-by-moment experience that both the yoga text and Tolle are speaking about. Give this a try next time you clean, wash the dishes, dust, iron, sweep, or do any other tedious task:

- Take a few breaths and feel your feet on the floor.
- Scope out what needs to be done.
- Pick a place to begin.
- With each movement, watch how the object you are cleaning changes.
- Notice the state of your body. If you are uncomfortable, shift your alignment.
- If you find your awareness drifting away, reset your attention to what you are doing.
- Continue to notice each step of the process until you finish.
- Now, look at the end result and notice the changes.
- Check in and become aware of how you feel.

When you bring this deeper level of awareness to your activities, you will notice how much more there is to appreciate throughout your day. The smallest shift will open you to a variety of opportunities that enrich and uplift your life in a way that you could not imagine. Even if you choose not to iron, go out and embrace your day—wrinkles and all!

WEEK THIRTY-NINE

HABITS

Daily living is deeply influenced by our habits. In January you started with a clean slate for the New Year. You were hopeful that this year would be an exciting, uplifting time filled with new accomplishments. It is October and maybe you have accomplished much of what you anticipated, but some could have fallen by the wayside.

There is one thing that seems to prevent your dreams from becoming reality—your mind! Yes, the mind that you count on for advice, intellect, and infinite wisdom often distracts you. You do not even realize what your thoughts say and wonder why, after you have researched, planned, and put in great effort, you still fall back into the old behaviors. You try to take pleasure in your day-to-day living, only to be derailed by your thoughts.

It really does not matter whether you have to run errands, have tickets to a show, or are going on a dream vacation (my personal preference). One common denominator will impact your overall enjoyment—your habitual outlook on life, both in thought and word. Let me give you an example.

I once knew someone who used the word "terrible" to describe everything that she perceived as inconvenient in her life and the lives of others. Terrible can denote something that causes great fear, alarm, or dread; but this certainly does not match the reality of sorting through a pile of newspapers or getting a flat tire!

No matter what is going on in our lives, the language we use has a tremendous power over how much pleasure and satisfaction we bring into our day. Words carry tremendous power.

The documentary "What the Bleep Do We Know Anyway" focuses on the power of words and features Dr. Emoto, who performed studies on water. Using the written and spoken word, he found that water actually "changed expression" depending on the thoughts and feelings directed toward it. He said: "Thoughts and feelings affect physical reality. What we think and say impact our entire being."

There are many words we repeat constantly either out loud or to ourselves—swear words, little barbs, colloquialisms. Think of some that you say. Right now, you might be thinking: "So what does that have to do with my plans for the day, week, or year?" Rest assured, it will make a big difference.

Let's take a look at what yoga says about the mind. The text emphasizes that when the mind broods over a mantra, it becomes identified with it. (Stop here for a moment. What did you just think when you heard the word mantra? You have nothing to worry about; I will not have you chanting anytime soon!)

Mantras are sounds, syllables, words, or group of words that are capable of creating transformation. Think of mantras as Scrubbing Bubbles® for your mind, to help clean up the old vocabulary and thoughts that are no longer needed. There are countless mantras and every tradition has simple phrases from which to choose. It can be a short prayer or a word that you can repeat frequently.

There are many words we constantly repeat to ourselves. We repeat statements such as "I will never be able to do that," "My body is a mess," "I'm uncoordinated," or "I'm not that smart" among many examples. We not only reiterate them, we actually reflect on them, we take them out to dinner, and obsess on them. We are not just satisfied with one negative thought and word, we have many. These are mundane mantras and the mind gets stuck on them. The only transformation they create is changing upwelling joy and freedom into limitation and lack. This is not what the yoga text is referring to.

Our minds habitually think and say things to ourselves that fall into this category. No matter how brilliant and evolved we are, our minds still have limitations.

The texts of yoga and every other tradition refer to the "Higher Self" or "Universal Consciousness." Call it what you want, but in a nutshell this is the positive, calm, centered part of you and, yes, we all embody it— even those whom you dislike!

How do we change our ingrained habits? We need to start somewhere, so let's begin with the words we use. The first step is to realize you are saying it. You cannot transform what you are not aware of. There are reasons we are not conscious of what we are saying and I have touched on them throughout the previous weeks:

- We have had years of conditioning and are oblivious to what we are saying.
- We are not in the moment because we are in reaction.
- Our minds are busy thinking ahead, not listening to others.

My student reports that when she gets excited or has a thought, before she knows it the words have departed from her mouth and are replaced by her foot! Her wise children say: "Mom, where is your filter?"

To change the words you use:

- First, you need to be aware of the need to change and see the effect your words have.
- You must have the desire to change.
- Have an idea of what words you can use to replace the old words to convey what you mean. Then you will know how to use them.

How do we accomplish this change? The first step is: Slow Down! Not so easy, but it can be done.

- Take a breath. (Yes, I am saying that over and over—a new mantra!)
- Listen carefully to what you are saying while you are saying it.
- Identify someone in your life who you can ask to gently help you notice what you are saying. For example, did you mean *terrible*? That is not an opportunity for commentary on your every word, but when you have a habit of using a particular word, having someone point it out will help you become aware.
- To begin cultivating the habit of more positive thoughts, try using a mantra that you are comfortable with from your own tradition. Some examples are *Soham,* (pronounced So'Hum, means "I Am"), *Om* (can be thought of as union of body, mind, and spirit), *Om Shalom* ("peace"), Namaste ("I honor the divine within"), and Peace.

Once you begin to notice the words you use, you will catch yourself after you have said or thought them. This is a positive step, even though it might not feel good. You have made a beginning. Do not use that as a reason to beat up on yourself (although, that would give you an opportunity to notice your unconstructive words!). Some of us have been using negative words and thoughts for decades. Habits take time to change so dedication is needed.

There is a payoff for your perseverance. Your negative mantras will dissolve and you will find yourself looking through a more positive lens at your daily activities. Find some new mantras that are uplifting and supportive of all that you want and deserve in life.

WEEK FORTY

PROCRASTINATION

I felt the topic of procrastination was pertinent to daily living but as I tried to write this section I found that I was dragging my feet on getting started. (Hmmm, maybe I needed to read this one.) We explored habits in Week Thirty-Nine, and procrastination falls into that category. It is problematic for many of us and we have been struggling with it for years. First let's take a look at what makes us procrastinate.

The Artist Way, by Julia Cameron, discusses the spiritual path to higher creativity. Creativity not only applies to the arts, but anything we are trying to produce. I have included a few excerpts from her book that are pertinent to procrastination:

> This kind of look-at-the-big picture thinking ignores the fact that a creative life is grounded on many, many small steps and very, very few large leaps.

> Rather than take a scary baby step toward our dreams, we rush to the edge of the cliff and then stand there, quaking, saying, "I can't leap. I can't. I can't..."

In Week Two, I wrote about discipline, perseverance, and the concept of one day at a time. Now, we need to simplify even more. Accomplish your project one minute, one simple task at a time; otherwise we will sabotage what we know we want to achieve. In many circles the acronym KISS is used —Keep It Simple Sweetie. (I know many use the word Stupid, but I get no inspiration from that.)

I am aware that the process of moving forward can feel daunting, but action is the antidote. A friend of mine used the analogy of conquering the fear of flying. She said, "Fly scared." Yes, we need to fly scared; moment by moment, step by step, until the big picture comes to fruition.

Most blocked creatives have an active addiction to anxiety. We prefer the low-grade pain and occasional heart-stopping panic attack to the drudgery of small and simple daily steps in the right direction....

In her book, Julie Cameron describes the fight-or-flight response that we looked at earlier, and we are clear that it wreaks havoc on our body and mind. Some of us are addicted to this rush, yet there is a cost to living this way. There are also times when we simply do not like what we must get done. (My husband wins the procrastination prize for not fixing the faucet, and he used to install plumbing as a job.) What we fail to realize is that when we postpone what we need to accomplish, it is still on our minds, creating tension for ourselves and everyone around us.

We must work with what we have rather than languish in complaints over what we have not.

This last point is at the heart of what keeps us stuck. We cannot be great at everything and often use our weaknesses as excuses to quit, rather than cultivate our strong points. Let me give you an example. When I began to write this book, I knew that my strength is not writing. My children and husband have a sophisticated command of the English language that I lack. I almost quit before I began, until my wise advisor reminded me that there are trained professionals who can fill in where I lack skill. What I do possess is knowledge and experience of the practices and philosophies contained in this book. I also have my own style of effectively communicating concepts that stay true to my voice and those I want to reach. As I continue to forge forward, I dive in deeper and hone the skills that are already inherent within.

There are always options available to us. We can get help or hire someone to do the parts that either we do not want to do or are incapable of accomplishing, so the only thing that holds us back is fear.

The main ally to procrastination is fear and it shows up in many forms:

We fear that we will never finish: If we keep our focus on the enormity of what we are doing, then we are sure to put if off indefinitely. There is a yoga teaching about this. It talks about the inner obstacles that distract us, and they stem from our minds. When we run up against an obstacle, we self-sabotage and slide back from the progress we have already made. When we understand we cannot always function on the same level and are able to let go of judgment, there will be room for the ups and downs of the process.

We fear reality: We are slow at following up on things that need our attention, such as preparing tax returns, studying for an exam, or returning a phone call. We know we need to finish, but we really want to avoid the outcome. We live by the rule, "what we don't know won't hurt us." Actually, it does because we carry the extra baggage of undone tasks and it weighs up down.

We fear that we never measure up: We think we will not do well, so why bother? We tell ourselves it is better not to try than to fail—emotionally that feels safer. We are left in the comfort of "less than" and take that attitude into our daily activities.

We fear success: In her book *Return to Love*, Marianne Williamson said, "Our deepest fear is not that we are inadequate. Our deepest fear is that we are powerful beyond measure. It is our light, not our darkness, that most frightens us." What we do not realize is that once we push through an obstacle (no matter how small), we gain a deeper understanding of our own capacity and pierce through to the next level.

There are a few things that I found helpful that will work for anything you want to accomplish:

- Guidance: Find someone who can help you—you cannot do everything on our own.
- Structure: Due dates and a step-by-step process (there can be some flexibility here) are vital.
- Positive people: Surround yourself with those who are supportive.
- Accountability: Find someone who can help you put together a time-line, and then report your progress. It can be the person you hire to give you guidance or someone else who is structured.
- Keep it simple: Easy, step-by-step, bite size pieces will work most effectively.
- Know your strengths: Focus on what feels more natural for you and then decide if you need accountability or someone else to help with the rest.
- Stay in the moment: When your mind drifts into fear, use any of the suggested practices to bring yourself back.
- Praise: Each step of the way, give yourself a pat on the back (or your shoulder if you can't reach your back) for beginning. Reward yourself in some small way.

Life is meant to be enjoyed and taking baby steps will transform your procrastination to momentum, and replace fear and anxiety with a sense of inner freedom. One final note—after completing this entry I felt relieved and happy and am now free to indulge in a well-deserved pedicure. Goodbye procrastination, hello relaxation!

NOVEMBER

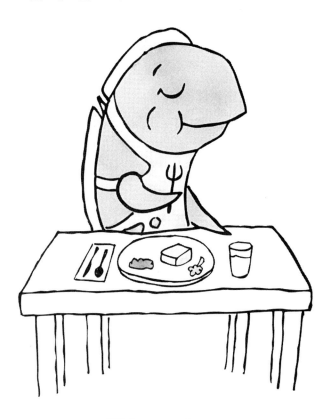

Digestion

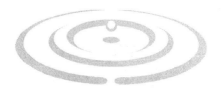

C U S T O M   C A L M

WEEK FORTY-ONE

FOOD GLORIOUS FOOD

There is an abundance of cooking shows on television and I appreciate the skill and creativity involved in preparing succulent dishes. (I live vicariously.) So much preparation is needed: from shopping for ingredients to setting the table. After all, we want our food to be attractive to look at before we take our first bite.

There are also popular food programs about racing to stuff down rich, unhealthy foods within a set time limit in front of a cheering squad. (I find these a bit scary.) Those shows bring to mind a well-known tune from the musical *Oliver*: "Food, Glorious Food." It is a playful song, sung by a group of poor, hungry orphans imagining an abundance of food; but in our country many of us eat our way into indigestion. November marks the onset of holiday celebrations. We spend time with friends, family, or co-workers with a drink in one hand and food in the other, as we simultaneously chat and nibble, unaware of what we are eating and drinking.

Thanksgiving and other holidays revolve around food. We spend hours shopping, cooking, planning, and decorating for the long-awaited feast. We sit down to a plethora of sides, entrees, and desserts, surrounded by friends and family. (Some of whom give you indigestion without taking a single bite!)

Now it is time to eat. We scarf down the food and before we know it we feel boated, uncomfortable, and ready for a nap. What happened? Did we really taste the food or only the first bite? We over-ate without even realizing that we were full.

Many articles about overeating give some insightful solutions. The *New York Times* ran an article entitled "Mindful Eating as Food for Thought." It addresses how we can enhance the experience of eating by being aware of the food as well as how the body feels.

We touched on mindfulness earlier in the book, but now let's take a look at what mindfulness really means. Jon Kabat-Zinn, one of the pioneers of mindfulness states "Mindfulness means paying attention in a particular way; on purpose, in the present moment, and nonjudgmentally."

The term "mindful eating" seems kind of uninviting, so I will make it a bit more enticing. When you are present with what you are eating you will take delight in your food, eat less, and feel more satisfied. So you are not dieting (do I have your interest now?), but rather enhancing your relationship to food.

Here are a few examples that illustrate this point:

I had recent dental work and one side of my mouth was quite sensitive, so eating became quite challenging. I was at a meeting and spotted one of my old time favorite cookies, the Vienna Finger®. I wanted one but since they are crunchy I hesitated to indulge myself, but soon gave into the temptation.

I took one and began eating by taking the sandwich apart and spreading the cream around. I proceeded to nibble away very slowly, savoring every bite. I hardly chewed and just let it melt in my mouth. I realized in my slow, mindful eating of the cookie I enjoyed every crumb. I normally would have eaten at least two (okay four) cookies in the time I took to eat just one.

When I was training with Jon Kabat-Zinn, we participated in 36 hours of silence. This included no music, no eye contact, no shopping, no phones, no writing, no hobbies, or reading (I admit I cheated and read the road signs and t-shirts.) I had some concerns about my ability to complete this assignment. When it came time to eat, I slowly selected my food and arranged it on my plate in a way that appealed to me. I carefully chose a picturesque view and sat down. Every morsel I ate tasted delicious. I could sense the texture, color, aroma, sound, and flavors, immersing myself in the entire process of eating. What I found most interesting was that I became aware that I was getting full and ate less than I normally would.

In both encounters I examined my relationship with food and how much more I enjoyed it when I was in the present moment. On both occasions I left feeling satisfied without overeating.

Eating gives us the opportunity to embrace and savor life. When you are aware of what you are eating, the flavors as well as the entire experience will intensify. Think of it as a form of meditation. (Yes, a new enticement to meditate). If you are dining with another person, and when you are not speaking, take a bite and enjoy it; then resume your conversation.

Take a few minutes and try this:

- Pick one type of food that you normally eat. It can be raisins, popcorn, chocolate, or some other snack.
- Take one piece and first feel the texture in your hand.
- Look at it on all sides.
- Smell it and take in the aroma.
- Now, take it to your lips and take a small bite, without chewing.
- Sense the flavor, texture, and the effect it is having on you as you roll it around in your mouth.
- Slowly chew it as you continue to experience the entire sensation associated with what you are eating. Include both your body and mind.
- Continue to finish the piece of food in this way and notice how you feel.

Next, try mindful eating at one meal.

> - Close the newspaper and turn off the television, cell phone, and music.
> - Set a place for yourself at the table.
> - When you sit down, first look at your food and engage your senses like you did when you practiced with the snack.
> - Now eat, and know you are eating as you take one bite at a time, while observing the response of your body and mind.

These principles are not easy to incorporate. I don't expect that many people will always be die-hard mindful eaters, but I invite you to incorporate these principles into your snacking and meals. As you slow down and become a bit more mindful of preparing and eating your food, you will feel satiated in a whole new way. Now that's some food for thought!

WEEK FORTY-TWO

THANKSGIVING

Let's look at the holiday where food is in the forefront—Thanksgiving. Most of us are familiar with its derivation but a brief review will be helpful. The Thanksgiving holiday began with the Native American Indians sharing a celebratory harvest feast with the colonists at Plymouth. The festivities lasted three days but because there were no ovens, the desserts were not part of the meal. (That could be a problem.) It was around two centuries later that President Lincoln proclaimed a national Thanksgiving Day to be held each November. (I guess at this point dessert was added as a concession for cutting back to only one day.)

When we think about the Thanksgiving holiday there are a few aspects to be investigated: physical digestion, gratitude, and Native American culture.

Digestion

Many people have digestion issues; but even if you aren't one of them, this time of year we tend to either overeat or eat richer foods than usual, resulting in some form of indigestion. Indigestion is a common complaint and often occurs because we are not aware that we are full. According to current information, it takes about ten minutes for our brain to register that we are satisfied, so when we eat quickly or are distracted, we do not realize that we are satiated until it is too late.

We already looked at mindful eating last week, so let's broaden our scope and include another cause of digestion issues. *The Wall Street Journal*'s March, 2009 article in *New Health Journal* addressed the effects of stress on our digestion.

L. Edwards, director of the Behavioral Chronic Pain Management program at Duke University Medical Center, said: "Now, we recognize that what happens in the brain affects the body and what happens in the body affects the brain." The article goes on to say:

> The digestive tract has its own extensive system of nerve cells lining the esophagus, stomach and intestines—known as the gut brain—that are extremely sensitive to thoughts and emotions. That's what creates the feeling of butterflies in the stomach. When anxiety persists, it can set off heartburn, indigestion and irritable-bowel syndrome, in which the normal movement of the colon gets out of rhythm, traps painful gas and alternates between diarrhea and constipation.

This is not a pretty picture, but it is the truth. I know I sound like a broken record about the impact of stress, but I am not making this up. I realize that most of us acknowledge that stress has an effect, but it is greater than we imagine.

Stress produces tension in our internal organs, decreasing their oxygen supply. This directly influences our ability to take in nutrients from food. The more oxygen that is absorbed in our internal organs, the healthier they are. We definitely want to keep our internal organs happy.

All of the techniques and perspectives explored in earlier chapters help temper stress. In addition, yoga practices are beneficial.

Specific yoga poses help with this because they give internal organs a massage, which brings in more blood and oxygen. The form I teach helps to decompress spinal tension, alleviating pressure on the organs, which helps augment blood supply. Find a practice that is right for you. Remember, yoga is to be practiced slowly and mindfully and always remember to check in with the wisdom of your body.

There is a simple yoga pose that helps relieve bloating and gas. It is fondly known as the Wind Relieving Pose. I would recommend waiting at least a half hour after a big meal before practicing this or any form of exercise.

I will give simple instructions but if you are confused or uncomfortable, wait until you work with a skilled instructor.

- Lie on your back with your legs together, and your lower legs over a blanket or chair; or simply keep your knees bent with your feet side by side.
- Bring both knees to your chest and bring hands over to the left knee, and replace your right leg back over the blanket or back to the floor. Keep it close to the midline of your body.
- Leave your right leg where it is and support your left knee with your hands either near your kneecap, or behind the knee crease.
- Do not pull it in, but relax as you hold it. Keep it pointed toward your left ear. Stay here for a minute or two. Repeat on the other side.

This pose can be done in bed or on the floor. Another pose is Thunderbolt and it is one pose that is appropriate to practice right after eating to help digestion, although for many it strains the knees. When I teach the pose, I use a lot of props, so you really need to work directly with a skilled professional that will meet you where you are.

I will once again revert to the breath, because it provides many digestion benefits. The slower, deeper breath (see Week Thirty Three, three-part breath) creates movement in your diaphragm that massages your stomach and other organs, increasing oxygen flow and nutrient absorption as well as expediting the elimination of waste. In addition, there are more aggressive breathing practices that stimulate your digestive fire, but you must learn them in person from an experienced instructor.

Gratitude

We dove into the topic of gratitude in February and it is worth mentioning again. Thanksgiving is essentially about giving thanks (hence the name) but it seems to become a food-a-thon and stress inducer, and the icing on the cake (no pun intended) is the inevitable indigestion. Some families have a tradition of asking each person around the table to share what they are grateful for, which is a nice beginning, but does not go far enough. In many cases the gratitude is forced, said quickly, and can come across as kind of corny. Saying what you are thankful for and behaving with gratitude are two different things. This phrase applies: "Don't just talk the talk, but walk the walk." I remember when my children would apologize for the same thing over again, I would tell them: "Don't apologize; change your behavior." That did not go over well, as apologizing is much easier. It is the same that with gratitude. Refer back to Week Thirty One for ideas on how to cultivate gratitude in your life.

Native American Culture
In today's world there is great concern for our environment and the neglect and disregard it receives. We can learn a lot from the deep respect for Mother Earth and for all of creation embodied in Native American culture. This poem by Black Elk, from the Oglala Sioux tribe gives us a glimpse into the true essence of their traditions and philosophy:

>Peace...
>Comes within the souls of men
>When they realize their
>relationship, their oneness,
>with the universe
>and
>all its powers,
>and when they realize that
>at the center of the Universe
>dwells Wankan tanka,
>and
>that this center
>is really everywhere,
>It is
>within each of us.

Wankan tanka means "the sacred" or "the divine" and when we ponder the message of Thanksgiving, it is one of gratitude for all that is, all that has been, and all that will be. This is a way of life, the heart and soul, and the spiritual essence of the Thanksgiving holiday.

Keep this in mind and slowly savor your family and food and have gratitude for all the gifts in your life. If those at your table have overeaten, wait a bit and then guide them in the three-part breath slowly and easily. It can be the after dinner activity. Who knows, maybe you will be the pioneer of a new Thanksgiving tradition!

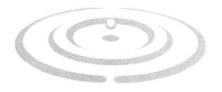

C U S T O M   C A L M

WEEK FORTY-THREE

CULTIVATING ATTITUDES

As we consider digestion, you would be shortchanged if I didn't dive deeper into what I feel is paramount to living a happy, fulfilling life. It is our capacity to assimilate, comprehend, and shape our experiences.

Our daily life is filled with challenges to understand and tolerate others' ways of behaving. This time of year we participate in festivities where we socialize with family, friends, acquaintances, and office staff; some of whom we would prefer not to spend time with. A significant factor that will help influence our capacity to absorb these events is whether we are accepting of others' personalities and beliefs.

History provides many examples of how attitudes and judgments of others have negatively influenced everyone involved. This brings to mind the popular Biblical story of Joseph. As the youngest son, he was closer to his father and the special treatment he received (including the coat of many colors) caused a good deal of tension and envy from his brothers. His dreams were powerful and this special gift generated even more jealousy, so the brothers devised a plan to get rid of Joseph. They sold him to the Egyptians. This story exemplifies the human condition of judging others based on our attitudes toward their talents, personalities, behaviors, and successes.

Maybe we have not sold someone we do not like into slavery, but I am sure we have had thoughts on how to get rid of those who bother us! Our lives, like Joseph's family, are affected by our perceptions, judgments, and behavior toward those who disturb us. The real problem arises when our attitude limits our ability to live a peaceful and centered life. It is part of the human condition, so if you are human you probably partake in some of these attitudes. Please do not berate yourself (or go into denial). Take this as an invitation to become conscious of thoughts you might not even know you have.

Every tradition offers help with this challenge. The yoga texts have some relevant philosophy and I broach this subject now because this time of year we need a little extra help. I usually introduce this concept to my students right before Thanksgiving and it is greatly appreciated.

The teaching tells us that the agitation in our mind stems from our thoughts and opinions of others. Most people we meet fall into four categories and when we cultivate certain positive attitudes toward them, our state of mind will remain calm and undisturbed.

Let's take a close look at the four attitudes:

Attitude #1: Cultivate friendliness toward the happy

Some people we know are happy about their successes and are filled with excitement and joy. However, before we know it, even as we are congratulating them, jealousy creeps in. This disturbs our state of mind, especially if we want for ourselves what they have attained.

Shifting your attitude to open up to their joy and celebrate their happiness can fill you up, leaving you feeling calm and centered.

Next time you feel uneasy around someone's happiness, take a breath and notice what is bothering you. Then bring yourself back to the moment and make the choice to shift your thoughts to an attitude of friendliness and happiness toward their success.

Attitude #2: Cultivate compassion for the unhappy

This one seems easy when we first look at it. Of course we are compassionate toward others who are not happy. However, we have all encountered people who are whiny and annoying and at times we would like to shake them and tell them to chill out! It is easy to get frustrated and judgmental toward those individuals.

When you find yourself feeling impatient with someone who is unhappy, even if their behavior is inappropriate, take a breath and look beyond the behavior and practice compassion even if you do not feel compassionate. This concept was considered in depth back in the February entries. What I can add here is one more aspect that I find most helpful. Recognize that those who are unhappy and negative are not at peace; realize how difficult and painful it must be to live that way.

Your shift in attitude from annoyance to compassion will calm your mind. Open up to looking beyond others' discontent and your judgment will slip away. I remember when my children would complain about someone else's inappropriate behavior, I would say; "Aren't you glad you don't have to behave that way? If they were happy, they would not act like that."

Remember, you can act with compassion while taking care of your needs around a negative, unhappy person. You will know you behaved with kindness and it will ripple throughout your day.

Attitude #3: Cultivate delight in the virtuous

I am sure you have come across a person who is quite intelligent or talented, or a wonderful athlete well-respected by others, or someone who might be generous and kind. No matter what positive qualities a person might possess, there are times when envy will set in as their mere presence makes us feel "less than." We try to find something about them to pull them down a notch. We might not even realize we do this, but subtle negative thoughts often surface.

This thinking only disturbs your state of mind. To help foster a peaceful mind, cultivate appreciation, and take pleasure in others' virtuous qualities.

Try to find delight in people you might envy by noticing their good qualities and consider cultivating those aspects within yourself. Focus on their kindness, generosity, or whatever quality they display and practice emulating it. I remember I was told years back to make a list of what qualities I wanted in my relationships. I easily jotted down many that I deemed important. Then I was told, "Now, go and become them." Not easy, but true.

Attitude #4: Cultivate disregard toward the wicked

We have all come in contact with those who are rude, disrespectful, or downright mean. Why wouldn't we become defensive and judgmental? After all, we would never behave that way!

We touched upon back in Week Twenty Five. These people disturb our state of mind and emotions. It is helpful to keep a few important concepts in mind:

- Remember that you have had times when your behavior was inappropriate and harmful toward others.
- Do not take the person's behavior personally, even it is directed toward you. They did not wake up that morning and specifically pick you out to be rude to, even if it feels that way. Keeping this distance helps you ignore the behavior of others, which will make your life much more serene.
- Keep your focus on your feelings and responses, not theirs. That is the one thing you can control.

Throughout the holiday season notice your reactions to others. See if you can put the person you are struggling with in one of these four categories. Were you able to cultivate any of the attitudes? Did your state of mind change? Remember, this practice if for you. You are cultivating a more peaceful, joyous way of living with the capacity to digest your life experiences with a new perspective.

WEEK FORTY-FOUR

DIGESTING LIFE: DANA'S STORY

This inspiring story from one of my students really shows how to digest life on life's terms. It is an honor to participate in her incredible journey.

In Atlanta on June 2010, I was diagnosed with Stage IV non-small cell lung cancer, which is considered terminal and inoperable. The presumption is that **only** smokers can be diagnosed with lung cancer. Wrong—I've never smoked! There was no bad habit to kick to the curb, as I had not even started one! Now, there's some food for thought.

Imagine being diagnosed with lung cancer at age 49, not having had any other illness except for a dry cough for a month and occasional bronchitis. Since I had been working like crazy, I figured that's why I was so tired and had lost 10 pounds over the winter. Next thing I knew, I was admitted to the Intensive Care Unit in critical condition with fluid filling the left lung, and massive pulmonary embolisms/blood clots! As they drained fluid off, the technician collapsed my lung! Wow, talk about intense pain! That day qualified as the first of many requiring major digesting of life's challenges!

Following a week of hospitalization, I was released with a diagnosis of pulmonary embolisms and pneumonia. At the follow-up appointment, I was blindsided and told I also had the "C" diagnosis. How does one explain that?

I acknowledged the seriousness of this situation by traveling to Michigan to be near my family and friends for support on the difficult journey ahead. Because I wanted to create a more positive spin on things, I asked everyone to now refer to my treatment plan as "Sunshine." I needed the affirmative imagery to help digest all the grueling treatments to come.

During two more July hospitalizations in Michigan, my oncologist offered participation in a clinical trial for mass infusions of Vitamin D, including mega doses of "Sunshine." Know what sunshine is also associated with? Vitamin D! Was that synchronicity or what? You betcha I joined the trial. No indigestion that day!

Scans showed that the cancer had metastasized through to the bone, especially in my back/sacrum which caused the intense bone pain I was now experiencing.

During that summer I focused on keeping my immune system protected; reading meaningful books, using affirmative language, practicing guided imagery, meditating, and repeating mantras.

Aside from the treatment itself, the biggest challenge was being away from the familiarity of my own home in Atlanta and having to stay away from my beloved cat, too, because he might potentially compromise my immune system further. To have all of my biggest creature comforts in life taken away at this critical juncture was beyond difficult. At times I reflect back and wonder what got me through. The steadfast will to live and refusal to give up certainly factored in there, as well as self-advocating through the medical and insurance maze, along with many good vibes, positive thoughts, and well wishes from loved ones.

In mid-September, I finished all four rounds of "initial treatment" with a slightly shrunken main lung tumor. I struggled with daily life at this point, as I could barely sit, walk, stand, lie down, or eat like a "normal" person would. Finally, in October I had five rounds of radiation to my sacrum only, since the back pain continued to intensify. I decided from day one though, that I while I had lung cancer, it wouldn't have me; even at this stage, despite what those around me were thinking!

Now back in Georgia, I had no one assisting me with daily activities, but at least I was home in a peaceful quiet environment, which intuitively I knew was critical for my continued healing. For most of the next 10 months, I just sat in a recliner, doing nothing. Eventually, I found a new local doctor, had additional testing, was diagnosed with a known lung cancer mutation and began taking a "targeted therapy" cancer drug. That drug is still saving my life along with daily injections to my stomach (yes, it hurts!!) to prevent future embolisms.

Then life's path changed again! I found an incredible cancer wellness program in Atlanta, which is where I began a journey back to better health, despite having lung cancer. I threw myself into weekly sessions of yoga, Pilates, wellness workouts, tai chi, mindfulness, and cooking demonstrations.

Through these courses, I've come to learn some interesting lessons regarding digestion:

- Staying "grounded" while commuting in Atlanta traffic—a major accomplishment.
- While sitting in Congressional offices during a Capitol Hill lobbying visit, riding the wave of pain from prescription side effects was a challenge to overcome!
- Remaining "present and in the moment" while I await my CT scan results every 90 days reduces stress and helps keep that "scanxiety" away.
- Riding the wave of nerves from packing for travel was a lesson learned in mind over matter.
- Mindful practices to still my thoughts and reduce questions of "what if" keep me "centered."
- Yoga and other practices to stretch my mind and my body thereby improving my overall health and have continued to give me "stable" results on every CT exam in the last year, for which I'm thankful. *Yay!*

The metaphor that best describes my journey seems to be that of an elastic band. We all know that an elastic band that is too tight can affect digestion. While admiring my new yoga pants, I realized that just 18 months earlier, I literally could not wear anything with an elastic waist, because it hurt my back too much from the metastasis mentioned earlier. Now here I was, feeling healthy, calm, renewed, less stressed, and happier. I felt as if I had sprung back to life in my new pants, much of which I attribute to the many life lessons I had learned from all the mind/body work that had become so meaningful. Remarkable for a Stage IV survivor!

Here's a final thought to chew on: If you have two lungs, you are at risk for lung cancer. In honor of the month of November, please join me in supporting National Lung Cancer Awareness month. You might not know this, but lung cancer kills 160,000 Americans every year, and it is the #1 killer from all cancer deaths, of both men and women. Just say "no more" to lung cancer. I am well.

Dana's message is clear. Her story is one of hope, empowerment, and choice. She embraces life fully and draws on life-enhancing practices to support her incredible journey. One final note—Dana just returned from a check-up and reported that they saw *no* evidence of lung cancer. Now that is something to digest!

DECEMBER

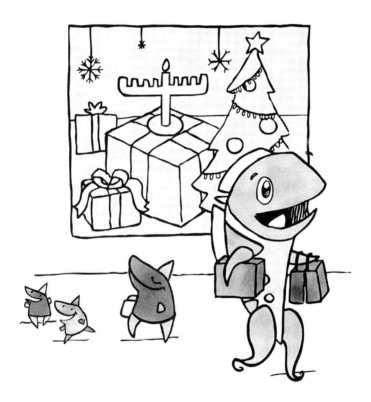

Stress

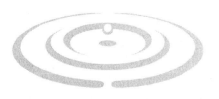

CUSTOM CALM

WEEK FORTY-FIVE

ENJOY THE HOLIDAY SEASON

Take 1

It is that time of year again. We wake up in the morning with excitement and anticipation of sharing our holiday cheer with the world. We look forward to the Christmas jingles, the holiday decorations, the opportunity to give, and the purchase of those special gifts for the people we love. It is the season of celebrating miracles, birth, and the end of year—we wish it would never end.

Take 2

Oh my, it is that time of year again. Traffic, crazy drivers, packed shopping malls, holiday decorating, relatives, year-end deadlines, and debt. If I watch one more commercial (it has been months; haven't we suffered enough?) or hear one more holiday song, I will scream. I wish it would end!

Take 3

The reality: Whether you celebrate the holidays or not, your comfortable, well-paced routine is thrown by the wayside. Stress is a fact of life and during this time of year it is magnified by the increase in commitments both at home and work. We find that even the fun and exciting times in life are stressful. The question is: How do we experience it all and diminish the symptoms of anxiety and fatigue that surface?

Let's look at a few common issues and how you can intervene and throw yourself a life preserver.

Shopping

Unless you sit in your house and order every gift and grocery item on the Internet (a good thought, but not practical), you will have to venture out and spend time shopping. Let's begin with the mall or any department store. (In case of emergency overwhelm, check for the nearest exit when you arrive!) You walk in and are inundated with decorations and crowds, which can feel quite intense. With it all, there is an opportunity to participate in the holiday spirit and your success will be determined by where your attention lies.

You have a few options: You can either try to muscle you way through and get your shopping over with (this imparts a Grinch-like attitude), or you can slow down and enjoy the process. The reality is, resistance is futile—you will wait in line or bump into others whether you want to or not, so why not go with the flow? Let me be clear, slowing down does not mean passing up partaking in holiday events. What it means is that while you are participating, you are present.

In Week Forty-One one of the techniques discussed was mindful eating. Now let's focus on mindful shopping. Rather than rushing through your shopping, take a moment to stand still and look at the decorations, people, colors, and designs. You can take a minute to consider the process of making the products, the abundance of the earth, the talent of creative minds, and the intelligence of business people and logisticians to get the products to us. There is so much happening around us that can be uplifting if we allow ourselves to become immersed in the experience.

Memory

When you finish your shopping, you go to meet a friend for lunch. In the frenzy of the crowded parking lot, you have forgotten where you left your vehicle. Even the wreath and reindeer antlers you attached to your car are of no help! You try your key fob but you are too far away to hear the gentle beep you are listening for. Your enjoyable outing ends with frustration and frenzy as you look for a security guard to help you out. Sound familiar?

I was watching a show on memory and the host said that anyone's memory can improve. As they showed one technique, I realized that a lot of what they were talking about was paying close attention. Only in the moment can you stay aware of what is happening around you. (Okay, writing it down helps too.)

When you park the car, you are already thinking about what you need to do next and you are on your way, before even looking at markers that will tell you where your car is.

The following practice helps me when I am out and about:

- Get out of the car.
- Stand still and take a breath.
- Look around and find something that will remind you where you are parked (another car would not be a good idea) and bring your focus to that reminder for a few seconds.
- Walk toward you destination and notice where you are and what you are passing as you do this.
- If you are taking an elevator from a parking deck, notice which side the elevators are on, which direction you turned and where you are entering.

You can use this technique throughout your day. The key is to stay present with what you are doing at that moment. It takes time to make this shift, so start with easy things, like your coffee mug or cell phone. (These are my top two.)

Recharge

After you have spent the day working and shopping, you are tired but you have a commitment that evening. You only have a short time to relax and need to make the most of it. A few minutes with your legs up the wall will quickly help you to restore and recover. It is also beneficial for varicose veins and circulation, as well as providing new blood flow to your upper body.

Try this:

- Lie on your back with your butt about 6 to 12 inches away from the wall. Bring your legs to the wall.
- Allow your head to be level. If it is not, place a pillow or towel under your head.
- Bring your legs side by side with your heels close to each other against the wall.
- Allow your knees to straighten with your thighs relaxed (if they are not, move further from wall). Do not lock your knees.
- Take easy breaths with your belly relaxed for a few minutes. You can use any of the breathing techniques from previous chapters.

Do not do this if you have detached retina, glaucoma, or hiatal hernia. Also, if your knees hyperextend (extend back creating pressure), place blankets behind your hamstrings to take the pressure off your knees.

This season will go so much smoother when you take pleasure in shopping, you easily locate your car, and indulge in some down time. My wish for you is to embody the themes of Christmas and Hanukah (as well as the chocolate). Give birth to a relaxed way of being and enjoy the miracle inherent in sharing your inner light with everyone around you. It is the gift that keeps giving. Happy Holidays!

WEEK FORTY-SIX

THE TRUTH ABOUT STRESS

As you have gathered from the emphasis in this book, stress is a fact of life. Many use stress as their driving force. A January 24, 2012, *Wall Street Journal* article looked at the positive influences that non-harmful stress can have. The feeling of being pumped up a bit and excited in a positive way can increase blood flow to the brain and limbs. Athletes use this kind of pumping up to make them more effective. However (I am sure you knew that was coming), sometimes we are unable to turn it off. Stress envelops us, producing harmful consequences to our health. You know the feeling. You get dizzy, angry, and loud. Your blood rushes, your heart beats erratically (okay not all at the same time or you would be on your way to the hospital) and more.

Martin Rossman, a clinical instructor at the University of California, San Francisco, Medical School explains:

> People under harmful stress lose the ability to re-engage the parasympathetic nervous system, which drives the body's day-to-day natural functions, including digestion and sleep. While individuals vary in how long they can tolerate chronic stress, research shows it sharply increases the risk of insomnia, chronic disease, and early death.

Emory and other universities have added yoga as a course for freshman. They are using yoga as a way to help students with stress and time management. The practice helps them prepare to handle the lifelong challenges of stressful situations. I venture to say that many of us would not need the information here if we had taken this course when we were eighteen. Unfortunately, yoga is associated with difficult poses, but what it really teaches is flexibility in managing daily life.

Kelly Kinsella has a one-woman show called *When Thoughts Attack*, and she's getting rave reviews because so many people relate to her message. I know most of us have plenty of material to write a sequel (probably an entire series), which makes me wonder why it is so difficult to calm our crazy mind.

We try to be proactive through yoga, massage, meditation, and exercise so we are familiar with feelings of relaxation and stability, but before we know it we are blindsided by anxiety. Taking time for classes is helpful, but sooner or later we must go about our day. There are times we need a life preserver before we drown in the reactions of our mind. We need a few quickies (no, not that kind of quickie—it's not practical enough and this is a family book!) that we can count on to get immediate results.

Here are a few ways to achieve instant relaxation; these exercises have saved me on a daily basis:

Find Your Mountain

A mountain is sizable, stable, and majestic. It maintains consistency, even with the change of seasons and weather. The landscape on the mountain might alter, but the mountain remains solid. (You can equate this to a bad hair day!) Even if the mountain is judged in some way, it does not crumble or whine. You must remember that you have the qualities of a mountain, even when you are in the grip of tension or storms in your life.

At work, there are times that we need to get centered quickly but it must be unapparent to others. (So, getting on the floor in your business suit is off the list.) If you are on your way into an important meeting, finding your solid, secure, calm self is just beyond the surface of your thoughts.

Try this:

- Stand with your feet solidly in the floor.
- Feel the contact of your feet to the surface beneath you.
- Bring to mind the image of the mountain and the attributes it embodies.
- Take a close look at its solid structure: the sides, the top, the landscape.
- Take a few breaths while feeling the weight of your feet tethered into the earth.
- Now, imagine you are that mountain; regal, centered, and empowered, and take that into your day.

If you are not one for visualizations, then simply feel the attributes that the mountain embodies and draw those feelings within.

Breath

I have already spoken about breath and there are many different practices to choose from. The following counting breath will quickly foster a calm mind:

- Begin to notice your breath moving in and out through your nose.
- Start to count the number of seconds it takes you to inhale, without forcing the breath in any way.
- Count the number of seconds it takes you to exhale, without forcing the breath in any way.
- See if you can even out the breath on the inhalation and exhalation.
- Count the breaths between 4 to 8 rounds.

Remarkably simple and incredibly effective, this technique can be done anywhere, anytime.

Chair Twist

There are occasions when sedentary practices are not enough and we need something physical to help both our bodies and minds. Many of us spend a lot of time sitting, particularly when we are at the computer. We get lost in our work until our discomfort and ensuing reaction gets our attention.

The following chair twist is convenient and easy to do. It has the added benefit of gently wringing out your spine to help with back and neck stiffness while quieting the mind. When doing this stretch, it is important for it to be effortless. The concept "less is more" applies here—the easier you do this, the more effective it is.

Try this:

- Sit sideways in an armless chair, with the back of the chair to your left. (If an armchair, sit facing forward.)
- Place your hands on the chair back and lengthen your spine upward. (If you are in an armchair, place your left hand on the chair seat and the other hand on the outside of your left thigh near your knee).
- Use your arms for support so you can allow your spine to relax, letting your arms do the work. Level your shoulders. Lightly draw in your navel for stability.
- You will twist toward the left.
- Twist from the bottom up. First, twist your stomach and waist, then your ribs, shoulders, and finally your neck and head—if you can, bring your head back from jutting forward.
- Use your arms to twist and allow your spine to relax. Take a few breaths and then come out slowly.
- Breathe in between each phase of the twist.
- Now, do the right side.

If you have osteoporosis or osteopenia, find out from your doctor if it is okay to do any twists. Please, be cautious when practicing twists. Do not go to your full range. Less is more.

Think of these simple techniques as a quick zap to your "attacking thoughts." They are free and do not require any change of clothes and do not hurt (sorry for those of you who live by the no pain, no gain philosophy). They can be done anywhere and take less than three minutes. Now that's a deal!

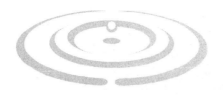

CUSTOM CALM

WEEK FORTY-SEVEN

RIDE THE WAVES: GREY'S STORY

My last entry highlighted some simple, effective centering tools that are easily applied in any situation. There is one more that has tremendous value, because it will change your entire experience of what precipitates stress. I feel safe to say, it will change your life—and I say this from experience.

I will introduce this with a story from an executive in a high-stress, corporate job.

> I work in a very stressful industry—financial services, specifically wealth management. I have been a broker/portfolio manager/financial advisor since 1985 so I have experienced some of the most stressful financial episodes since the Great Depression: the 1987 market crash, Iraqi invasion of Kuwait, the Tech bubble, 9/11, and the most recent financial crisis from 2007 to present. Clients rely on me to guide them through these tumultuous times and expect that I will not lose them any money (which of course is not realistic), and then they become quite upset when I report that their portfolio has declined by "x" percent. I have been called many obscene names and some have questioned my intelligence (one even implied that there might have some inbreeding in my family's past) so dealing with stress is paramount. Many people in my industry turn to alcohol, drugs, and other destructive activities that may ruin their career as well as their families.
>
> The market varies daily and it is easy to get derailed by the dramatic price fluctuations of a stock I might be following. The best way for me to deal with this is to stay in constant contact with the client and to be honest about the situation. I also walk around my

office and chat with other co-workers when we might commiserate about the day. This helps me realize that I'm not the only one suffering through difficult market conditions.

I tend to internalize many things, including stress, and then down the road I will explode at my wife or children for a small or insignificant thing that bothered me. But thankfully that doesn't happen very often so I don't have to sleep in the guest bedroom! As I have aged I have become more relaxed and forgiving of others and realize that life is too short to carry a chip on my shoulder.

I use sports and hobbies as a way to take my mind off whatever is bothering me. Somehow that StairMaster® makes a lot of worries go away as I reach the 100th floor of the building! I make sure to maintain "an even keel" in my personal and professional life so that stress doesn't get the best of me!

Grey's job requires him to follow the daily rise and fall of the stock market while remaining calm and precise. This is a great segue into the important concept of riding the waves. In March I spoke about pain and gave you information about the benefits inherent in anchoring your awareness in the present moment. We will now expand upon this as it relates to both stress and sensation.

Everything contains a wave—there is a beginning, a crest, and an ending. Our entire life is a wave: you are born, you peak, and eventually die. It is the same with breath, sound, sensation, thought, hot flashes (yes, there is an end), emotions, and fatigue.

Riding the wave is a foundational concept in many arenas, because it is based in awareness, not reaction.

When you learn to track the wave, your attention remains in the moment-by-moment experience, rather than on your reactions. Riding the wave of stress is essential to transforming it. When we have a stressor in life, there is the actual problem we are dealing with, but then we layer our thoughts, feelings, and emotions upon it, setting off a spiral of anxiety.

How do you take the emotional charge out of your experiences? The answer is simple, but not easy—you stay aware of every part of the occurrence. In other words, you track what is happening and when you do this, it diffuses your focus and takes the personalization out of it, as if you were reporting the news or weather.

Let's use a meteorologist's report as an example: *There will be rain and thunder tomorrow . . . oh my God, I was supposed to have my house painted . . . oh boy, now I have to reschedule and that is a real pain—I am so mad, my day is ruined!* This is how it would be if the reporter layered his emotions upon his report. (Hmmm, it could make the weather report quite entertaining). In actuality, the weather report is based on specific information (at times, misinformation), not feelings. I do not promise that it will not rain, but I can assure you that it is your reaction that propels the storms of your life, not actual events.

To begin to learn how to ride the wave of your reactions and thoughts try this:

- Focus your attention on the problematic situation and watch it without taking it personally, the way you would watch a weather report.
- As you watch, notice what is happening. Become aware of your thoughts—this includes your emotions and feelings as they arise from thoughts.
- Follow the wave of thought, without any opinions and judgments. Notice its beginning, middle, and end.
- Continue to do this with each thought.

To begin to cultivate riding the wave of sensation, try this:

- To begin with, avoid classifying your feeling as "pain." Instead, say "sensation."
- Find a place in your body where you notice sensation.
- Without using words to judge it or categorize it, simply track it and notice what you are feeling. For example, it might be a burning sensation that shifts into stinging or throbbing. It might move down your leg and pulse or feel hot or cold.
- Describe it factually, as if you were reporting the weather.
- Notice the sensation from the onset, to the crest, and through to its decline. You might have many sensations but each of them has movement when you really pay attention, even chronic sensations.
- You can softly direct your breath into the area you notice.

The efficacy of these techniques is based on evidence and as I said earlier, they are life-changing. You are in charge of shifting your reactions and it is not through force, but through your own awareness. Practicing this will save you from the negative consequences of stress and pain. I admit it takes time to integrate these practices, but it is worth the commitment. Imagine a life where stress and reactivity take a back seat to your full participation in a happier, healthier life. Ride the wave and guarantee yourself no wipeouts!

WEEK FORTY-EIGHT

SPLASH INTO CALM

When T.S. Eliot wrote "... the still point of the turning world" from *The Four Quartets* in 1943, he described what we so desperately need in our busy lives today: a sense of calm.

Activity does not need to stop for us to access inner calm and stillness. There seems to be some misunderstanding about this notion.

I was speaking with a friend who has a very full life and is always on the go. I asked her what her perception of calm was and she meekly said, "boring." We seem to think calm means that we are chilled out, laid back, and not stressed; that life is monotonous. That is far from the truth! You can live life calmly while having lots of energy; live where stress does not take you over, and enjoy what you are doing. Living a calm life means having the ability to roll with the punches, because life will assure you many punches.

Throughout this book, we have explored practices, techniques, and perspectives that you can easily integrate into your day-to-day living. They help you find your still point, beyond the chaos of the stressed-out mind (I promise, that calmness is there somewhere). In case you are still not convinced that a few minutes of practice a day can change your life, allow me to entice you with a review of a few of the many benefits. We need to know the perks of practicing these, or why bother? This is why:

Overall benefits of all centering practices:

- Improved relationship with your stress, pain, and illness, decreasing their impact on your life.
- Increased energy and vitality.
- Improved concentration, clarity, and memory.

- A stronger overall mental and emotional state.
- An understanding of your present experience and the way you react to it.
- The empowerment to immediately reduce your anxiety and stress.

Physical benefits:

- Improved sleep, more restful nights, and more comfortable, better days.
- Decreased muscle tension, allowing you to release and relax.
- A more stable heart rate.
- A more stable blood pressure.
- Improved digestion and increased physical comfort.
- Increased oxygen intake, enhancing brain and blood function and aiding overall well-being.
- Complementary and enriching to ongoing treatments for your pain, anxiety, and illness.

Benefits of breath:

- Brings you back to the moment, dissipating anxiety and fear.
- Stimulates the relaxation response, bringing you back from "fight-or-flight."
- Free and portable, usable in the very moment you face stress.

If these benefits do not convince you then you are one tough customer; but I can give you something more. Yes, the skeptic needs more proof beyond my word and the quotes throughout this book.

To convince yourself, I suggest you get on the Internet and type in "stress management articles" and read any of the six million hits that come up (they will either stress you out or help you sleep). An easier, shorter way is to just try a few techniques here and see for yourself.

There is so much to stress us out in the world. I remember years ago going to my internist for my ophthalmic migraines and he told me that he could give me medicine but thought they would go away on their own. He said, "Just do what you do" as a consultant, teacher, and yoga instructor, and they would probably stop. So, I "did what I do," which are the practices throughout this book, and sure enough, they went away.

I conceived of this book because I am a practical person who needs things kept very simple. I know I am in the majority with those who don't have a lot of extra time. Many of the professional trainings I have taken required practicing for an hour at a time, but the realist in me knows that I will not get my clients to do that. They would run the other way if I told them to do something for an hour—or even half an hour.

After years of experimenting, I realized that the short and simple techniques work the best. These practices are easy, non-intimidating, accessible, practical, free (except for the cost of this book or a few sessions), and effective. You do not have to believe or buy into anything. Take it day by day, weekly, or skip around to the topic that you need to learn about.

I would rather have my readers and clients be consistent for a few minutes a day than dive in and drift off, or worse, overdo it and burn out again. When the practice is short and simple, improvement is incremental, and one day you notice something has changed. That is when you really reap the benefits from the inside-out.

If, after reading these pages, you have an inkling of hope that you can live a life of calm while embracing each day, then I have been successful. In my heart, with total sincerity, I can say to you, *"If I can do this, anyone can."*

Pick a few favorite concepts or practices from this book and work with those until you feel comfortable. My personal favorites are: *Three Part Breath*; the phrase. *"This too shall pass,"* and *Riding the Wave*. All you need is an open mind and if you struggle with that, compassionately pry it open a bit each week (no pliers needed) so you can begin to learn how to take care of yourself. Reread this book each year and you are sure to uncover a new level of understanding and freedom.

A calm, stress-free, energized, productive, happy life is within your reach. All you need to do is practice! Splash into calm and enjoy every drop... *you deserve it.*

Bibliography

January
Week 2
> Susan Smith Jones, PhD, as quoted by Andy Zabko in *Treasury of Spiritual Wisdom*, San Diego: Blue Dove Press, 1996.

Week 3
> Quote by Leo Buscaglia (1924-1998). Author and professor, University of Southern California.
>
> Dr. Seuss. *Oh, the Places You'll Go!,* New York: Random House, Inc., 1960.

Week 4
> Quote by Robert L. Stevenson (1850-1894). Novelist, poet, essayist.

February
Week 5
> Quote by The Dalai Lama XIV.

Week 6
> Tom Sanders. *Love Is The Killer App: How To Win Business And Influence People*, New York: Crown Publishing, Inc., 2002.

Week 7
> Saki Santorelli. *Heal Thy Self*, New York: Three Rivers Press, 2000.

March
Week 9
> Jon Kabat-Zinn. *Wherever You Go, There You Are*, New York: Hyperion Publishing, 1994.
>
> Jessica Yadegaran. "In Yoga Class, Play it Safe," *Atlanta Journal Constitution,* February, 2012.

Quote by Henry Miller (1891-1980). American author and writer.

Week 10
Jim Carson and Kimberly Carson. Yoga of Awareness professional training, Duke University Integrative Medicine, 2007.

Quote by Hippocrates, 430 B.C.

Week 11
Camp Twitch and Shout, and Camp Sunshine, Twin Lakes Children's Camps. www.camptwinlakes.org.

Week 12
Institute of Medicine of The National Academics. *Relieving Pain in America,* June 2011.

Lauran Neergaard. The Associated Press, June 29, 2011.

Bravewell Collaborative. "Military to Implement Integrative Medicine for Comprehensive Pain Management," June 2011.

Craig Leibenson. *Rehabilitation of the Spine: A Practitioner's Manual,* Baltimore: Williams & Wilkins, 1996.

April
Week 13
E. Finzi and E. Wasserman. "Botox Injections," *Journal of Dermatologic Surgery,* 2006.

Amy Weintraub. *Yoga Skills for Therapists,* New York: W.W. Norton & Company, 2012.

Week 14
Quote by Joseph Campbell (1904-1987). American mythologist, writer, and lecturer.

Week 16
Quote by George I Guridieff (1866-1949). Russian spiritual teacher.

Chiam Potok. *My Name is Asher Lev,* New York: Random House, 1983.

Danna Faulds. *Go In and In and In,* Nebraska: Morris Publishing, 2002; permission granted.

May
Week 17
Rosalind Bentley "Just Too Ill to Chill," *Atlanta Journal Constitution,* May 15, 2011.

Week 19
Philip Chesterfield, as quoted by Andy Zabko in *Treasury of Spiritual Wisdom*, San Diego: Blue Dove Press, 1996.

Week 20
Quote by Stephen Levine. Poet, author, and teacher.

Mimi Swartz. "The Yoga Mogul," *The New York Times,* July 21, 2010.

Sri Swami Satchidananda. *The Yoga Sutras of Patanjali,* Virginia: Integral Yoga® Publications, 1978.

June
Week 21
Laura Landro. "The Hidden Benefits of Exercise," *The Wall Street Journal*, January 5, 2010.

Jane E. Brody. "Ancient Moves for Orthopedic Problems," *The New York Times*, August 1, 2011.

Chungliang Al Huang, as quoted by Andy Zabko in *Treasury of Spiritual Wisdom,* San Diego: Blue Dove Press, 1996.

Week 22
William Shakespeare, *Hamlet.*

Robert Fulghrum. *All I Really Need to Know I Learned in Kindergarten*, New York: Ballantine Books, 1986.

Albert Einstein as quoted by Andy Zabko in *Treasury of Spiritual Wisdo,*. San Diego: Blue Dove Press, 1996.

Week 24
>Quote by Charles R. Swindoll. Pastor, teacher, writer, president of Dallas Theological Seminary.

July

Week 25
>Quote by Gary Zukov. Noted author and teacher.

Week 27
>Dr. Gail Saltz. "Your Partner's Annoying Habits," *Today Show,* April 11, 2002.
>
>Quotes by Sally Kempton, interpretation, master yoga, meditation teacher.

Week 28
>Tina Fey. *Bossypants,* New York: Reagan Arthur Books, 2011.
>
>Lynn Peisner. "Child Anxiety Can Be a Big Issue," *The Atlanta Journal Constitution,* August 8, 2011.
>
>Rabbi Rami Shapiro. *The Sacred Art of Lovingkindness,* Vermont: SkyLight Paths Publishing, 2006.
>
>Laurie Goodstein. "Serenity Prayer Stirs Up Doubt: Who Wrote It?" *The New York Times,* July 11, 2008.

August

Week 29
>Quote by Albert Einstein (1879-1959).

Week 30
>Viktor Frankl. *Man's Search for Meaning,* Massachusetts: Beacon Press, 1946.
>
>Quote by Oprah Winfrey, talk show host, actress, philanthropist.
>
>Quote by Mayo Foundation for Medical Education and Research (1998-2012). www.mayoclinic.com.

Suzie Orman. "Change Your Attitude Before Changing Your Job," *Financial Disasters,* www.oprah.com, January 23, 2012.

Week 31
Helen Keller as quoted by Andy Zabko in *Treasury of Spiritual Wisdom*, San Diego: Blue Dove Press, 1996.

September
Week 34
Patrick Geraghty. "Combatting Cancer," *Sky Magazine,* June 2011, p. 129.

Week 35

Kelly Greene. "Caregiving Elders," *The Wall Street Journal*, June 4, 2011.

Helena Oliviero. "Caregiver's Anguish: I Need to be Two People," *The Atlanta Journal Constitution,* March 25, 2012.

Week 36
Quote by Eleanor Roosevelt (1884-1962).

Carolyn Leigh and Mark Charlap. Song title, I *Won't Grow Up,* BMI Carwin Music Inc., 1954.

Quote by Immanuel Kant (1724–1804), central figure in modern philosophy.

October
Week 38
Sri Swami Satchidananda. The *Yoga Sutras of Patanjali,* Virginia: Integral Yoga® Publications, 1978.

Eckhart Tolle. *The Power of Now: A Guide to Spiritual Enlightenment,* Canada: Namaste Publishing Inc., 1997.

Week 39
William Arntz, Betsy Chasse, and Marc Vicente. *What the Bleep Do We Know Anyway!?* Florida: Health Communications Inc., 2004.

Week 40
>   Julia Cameron. *The Artist's Way*, New York: Putnam's Sons, 1992, p. 142-143.
>
>   Marianne Williamson. *Return to Love*, New York: HarperCollins Publishers, Inc., 1992.

November
Week 41
>   Lionel Bart. Lyrics: *Food, Glorious Food,* London: Lakeview Music Publishing Company, Ltd., 1959.
>
>   Jeff Gordinier. "Mindful Eating as Food for Thought," *The New York Times,* February 7, 2012.
>
>   Quote by Jon Kabat-Zinn, PhD, founding director of Stress Reduction Clinic at University of Massachusetts Medical School.

Week 42
>   Melinda Beck. "Stress So Bad It Hurts," *The Wall Street Journal*, March 2009.
>
>   Black Elk, from the Oglala Sioux. *Catch the Whisper of the Wind,* Cheewa James Horizon Publishing, 2000; by permission.

December
Week 46
>   Sue Shellenbarger. "When Stress Is Good For You," *The Wall Street Journal,* January 24, 2012.
>
>   Jim Carson and Kimberly Carson. Yoga of Awareness professional training, Duke University Integrative Medicine, 2011.

Week 48
>   Quote by T.S. Eliot (1943). *The Four Quartets.*

About the Author

If you would have told me twenty years ago I would be teaching individuals and healthcare professionals skills to deal with stress, chronic illness, and pain, I would have asked to have my hearing checked.

How did I go from being in sales, an executive director, yoga studio owner, to CEO of Custom Calm, a coach, teacher, author, and speaker?

In one word, I would say "life" intervened. I have had many twists and turns in my life, which led me into the work I love and live.

I developed lupus after the birth of my younger daughter, and had chronic scoliosis pain. In my quest for avenues to help myself, I found gentle yoga and meditation quite beneficial. This led me to get advanced certification in gentle yoga and open a yoga studio.

Another life challenge came with my younger daughter's diagnosis of Dermatomyositis, a form Muscular Dystrophy (she is well now.) Yoga and meditation was helpful, but I needed to find a way to help myself stay calm in the midst of daily challenges.

I studied Mindful Based Stress Reduction techniques with Jon Kabat-Zinn of University of Massachusetts, and Awareness techniques at Duke Integrative Medicine. I coupled this work with my other trainings and business experience, to form Custom Calm, LLC. I love what I teach and am grateful for my journey.

I live in Atlanta, GA with my awesome husband Robert, and my quirky dog Kiddo. My adult children Jennifer and Jamie have moved to other cities and are busy building their own careers. Much like me, their past experiences shaped their work.

One thing I know for sure: If I can live calmly, so can you! Hope to meet you soon.

Warm Regards,
Ellen